BEHIND THE RED LINE

*An OR Nurse's Guide to Starting Out
and Succeeding in the Operating Room*

Contents

Title Page   1

Preface   5

Part One   9

    Chapter 1. Nursing School   11

    Chapter 2. OR Nurses Are Real Nurses   23

    Chapter 3. Making It In   43

    Chapter 4. Training   53

    Chapter 5. OR Culture   75

    Chapter 6. Teaching and Precepting   89

Part Two   107

    Chapter 1. The Smell of a Nurse in the Morning   109

    Chapter 2. Lace by the Fireplace   115

    Chapter 3. Birthday Cake   123

    Chapter 4. Last Fight   129

Preface

I am a full-time nurse in the operating room and have worked in multiple hospitals and roles in my career. The type of hospital work cultures out there are as numerous as the variety of work roles a nurse is called upon to do. I think I've worked long enough to get a good feel for nursing culture in the operating room, but I know my words won't convey the experiences every nurse, scrub tech, surgeon, or any other person in the OR have had. I can't tell the story of someone completely burned out from the job, or someone who has climbed all the way up the leadership ladder, although I've seen examples of both.

I can only write what I've seen and experienced to this point in my work life and what I think my perspective can offer to someone reading these pages. Ultimately it's a job, but one where we meet people at one of their most vulnerable moments, right before they have surgery. I wanted to write so that someone outside healthcare could understand what it is like from an OR nurse's perspective.

An OR nurse or someone else in healthcare will probably read many things they already know, but hopefully they can relate to what my experience has been. Whatever names appear in this book have been changed from their true identities. I am remaining anonymous because I felt I could more freely share my own experiences by doing so.

While writing, I have found this book has been somewhat for my own benefit since I have been able to deconstruct and reflect upon things that have happened to me that one can only do with hindsight. I want anyone curious about the OR whether they are about to enter nursing school, graduate, or thinking about switching their nursing specialty altogether to get a glimpse into a workplace that is not always discussed or promoted in nursing school. Many times the OR can be a misunderstood or intimidating place to those who have never been behind the red line. I hope after reading this book you will better understand what it's really like, at least from one person's point of view.

The industry itself and patients everywhere need good nurses in the operating room and I hope my words give curious readers a better idea of what it is like and become interested in possibly working there. Every nurse has "their people" - the specialties they've chosen and the reputations that surround them. I know ER nurses and oncology nurses that could write meaningful words about their places. This one is for the OR, and the masked people on the other side of the red line.

9

PART ONE

My Journey

Chapter 1. Nursing School

I will not take many pages to discuss the beginning of my nursing career. After all, this is a book about working in the operating room, and nursing school usually isn't a time for most nurses that we like to look back upon. However, I think it would be useful for you to know how I came to the place where I am now and why someone felt the urge to write a book about their job. Here in the beginning I will give you a look back from where I stand now in the job and how I became an operating room nurse. The destinations in nursing are endless, but the beginning is the same. The new grads all the way up to the chief nursing executives in the hospital all arose from the same place. We all started in nursing school.

After talking to several co-workers in the places I've been, I've found that the OR was a second or third nursing specialty for many. For others, the OR was where they landed after switching careers altogether. There are many paths nurses in all specialties have taken to get where they are, and the OR is no different. Along the way you will arrive at crossroads in your career, whether you make them appear yourself or they come out of nowhere. My own path had a few barriers and detours, but I eventually found myself where I am now.

I finished nursing school almost 15 years ago. My faculty was full of nurses with various backgrounds and various personalities. Some were retired but many were in active practice. The good ones taught you the necessary curriculum but also used their own life experiences from nursing practice to make their lessons stick. The poor ones had a "WELL, BACK IN MY DAY..." mentality and insinuated that you might not be cut out for nursing if they ever perceived you were unenthusiastic about something.

For these instructors there was a "gatekeeper" mentality and they wanted you to quit at the first sign of struggle. I can tell you what my experience was, but nursing schools seem to have changed as fast as some things about nursing itself, so I won't spend much time telling you how it used to be. I quite simply don't have a very contemporary perspective. I mention this though because from talking to some nursing students this mindset still exists. In my opinion, the work tasks and the learning itself does enough for the most part to "weed out" people that probably shouldn't be nurses.

A wise nursing instructor will recognize a struggling nursing student and determine if they should be encouraged to keep trying or if they should perhaps be advised to consider another field. Do not allow those people to discourage you however if you really want to pursue something. Persistence is an important trait to have in the OR, as I will tell you later.

Like much of formalized education today, nursing school prepares you very well for testing and things you need to know to graduate. The school you choose wants you to immediately start working in the healthcare industry after you graduate so they can tell prospective students interested in their programs that their students go on to get jobs in respected places. Little time is spent on finding the right place to go *for you*. I mean the hospital itself, but also the nursing specialty you land in. Some people are lucky enough to know where they want to go work before, during, and after nursing school. I was not one of these people.

The school's perspective is cut and dry: make the grades, show up to clinicals, graduate, and pass the NCLEX. It's up to you to know if you are really cut out for nursing. However, I do know that it is hard enough running a nursing school that gives the right balance of instruction, clinical experience, and preparation to pass the NCLEX. Nursing schools don't necessarily have the time to spend making sure students find their own niche.

I think it's best to explore as many perspectives as possible from the people themselves on the job. You will get advice from instructors if you ask, but nothing beats the honest voices of the nurses you meet. Talk to nurses you know with as many varieties of backgrounds as possible. A nurse on one floor in the hospital has completely different responsibilities than a nurse in another area. Sometimes the only common thing they have are the letters after the name on their badges. When it's time to start clinicals, get all the information you can from places you like and are interested in. If you find yourself in a place you definitely don't want to pursue, tough it out and learn all you can anyway. Remember what you learn because you never know when you may need that information again, and move on.

Nursing school generally prepares you for Med-Surg nursing. You get some ER, Pediatric, and OB clinical rotations, but mostly you have clinicals on the Med-Surg floors. These units have many common skills that you need to practice and are the bulk of nursing positions in the hospital. A good school gets you into a variety of places to see where you might fit in best after you graduate if you're unsure, and hopefully this includes some time in the OR.

Seeing as many places a nurse is capable of going will give you a well-rounded learning experience into things you may not get the chance to see very often. Working in the OR, we get the occasional nursing student visiting us on an observational clinical. It seems many of the nursing schools around me are good about at least getting the students one day in the OR; I've heard that some schools don't even bother. It's true that a nursing student cannot practice the limited skills they have during a clinical visit to the OR, but not letting them go at all is a significant disservice.

Even if the student already knows they want to go elsewhere when they finally earn the RN after their name, it isn't a wasted clinical to see the place where their trauma patient in the ER goes in order to get life-saving care. The orthopedic floor nurse needs to see at least once how the new knee or hip replacement their patients received were performed surgically. There are incredible things that happened in the OR underneath the stitches and surgical dressings. All nursing students should get the chance to see the advancements modern surgery has made and continues to make.

Obviously, the medical content in nursing school is absolutely necessary to learn. Yes, you need to buy the 1,000 page textbooks every semester. There is also something lacking though that I think nursing schools should attempt to convey to their students while they are still under their watch. In the final year of nursing school, there should be a class where students are made to dress in work attire and perform various nursing tasks.

Clinicals do not really accomplish this because they can

be very limited. You get to defer to the actual nurse when you cannot answer a question or need to do something that is outside of your scope of practice. The first thing you or the real nurse tells the patients is that you aren't a nurse! When the patient asks you something you didn't read in a textbook, you go ask the real nurse and slink off to the break room to nibble on graham crackers and question your decision of going to nursing school altogether. A nursing student on a clinical only experiences a fraction of what a fully qualified nurse does in their every day work. Clinicals of course have their place and a student's involvement is rightfully limited, but more is needed.

What I am talking about is training that prepares you, or at least gives a glimpse of what a hospital workplace can be like. There is a distinction between performing tasks and experiencing the workplace. Anyone can do a patient assessment in a training lab studying and practicing with fellow students that are coaching you along.

What is it that I suggest? A nursing student needs to find out what it's like to stand on your feet for almost all of a work shift and not go to the bathroom. As much as possible, give the nursing student a stiff dose of reality. Give them a long hallway with 6-8 rooms. The nurse gets a rolling computer station. In each room there is a person, ideally someone the student has never met, who is their "patient." Get volunteer students from other majors, nursing students that are about to graduate, parents, other professors, etc. Don't bother getting them to diagnose a disease or identify a symptom of an impending medical emergency. This is all about experiencing "real life."

One or two patients are "easy," but only to lure the student into a false sense of self-confidence. Get a few of the patients to be rowdy. I'm talking, get someone to throw a foley catheter with yellow colored water out into hallway and begin screaming their head off. Have another patient yell "HELP!" over and over. Get a patient's "spouse" to lean out into the hallway and give a disapproving look at the nurse. Have someone pour a full cup of soda on the hallway floor and don't tell the nurse about it, and don't send someone to clean it up. Make them decide how to handle it. Give the student nurse a work cell phone that rings steadily over the course of the training period. Let the phone be silent for half an hour, but then give them three or four calls in a row that require either a call to a physician or vigorous notetaking. Ideally this would occur while in a contact room or while helping a patient walk to the bathroom. Have another "nurse" leaning against the wall in the hallway faced down looking at their personal phone or taking a selfie while the learner is drowning. Hospital executives might frown on these ideas as it may sound as though I am criticizing the workplace. Trust me, it is this bad, and much worse sometimes. Even a good nursing floor will still have these things, but with redeeming qualities such as helpful co-workers, involved management, and a fully-staffed unit. Too many places though lack one or all of these traits.

Make this training hell, but make it passable. Give them a nursing assistant to delegate appropriate things to and a charge nurse to bail them out, but only a few times. This exercise should be at least four hours long. For every minute they sit down, they have a point deducted. Get them to talk about the experience after it's done. If this experience sounds too much for one person, get a group of four and give each person a one hour turn, the other three have to watch in silence as the nurse does their work. You must get them unnerved for this little period of time, but spend as much time at the end talking through what happened and encouraging them in a debrief session. I am just making suggestions. I think something like this would help prepare people better for what they might face after leaving nursing school. The medical concepts a nurse has to know are indeed hard enough to learn and practice. However, the personal interactions and unending work tasks are things that have to be experienced, not read about.

I will describe a little of what encapsulates being a floor nurse since so many new grads start there and that is the place where most nursing students spend a good many clinicals. Even I spent almost two years on a Med-Surg floor in the beginning of my career before finally getting into the OR. Floor nurses as they are collectively called if they work in Med-Surg have numerous responsibilities and demands. A great work day for them is when their patients are all on the way to improving and getting discharged, they have a good nursing assistant, the rest of the unit is fully staffed and they get to sit down for lunch. They even get to leave work on time!

A typical day will include a co-worker calling out absent, which creates more work for everyone. A patient might develop an emergent situation which requires their complete attention while other patients yell at them from down the hall for not getting them more crackers and soda. Work tasks that arrive in a constant stream that doesn't let them sit down for several hours. That patient's spouse who wanted the crackers and soda makes a complaint to the nurse manager for ignoring them. Meanwhile the nurse was trying to keep another patient alive...and sometimes the manager will take the other person's side!

Sadly a floor nurse might endure all of these things for years with no belief that things will get better. Eventually many succumb to "burnout." Seeing this burnout in many nurses in clinical after clinical as a nursing student was pretty discouraging. Some of the nurses looked like they were about to take a long drag on a cigarette and walk out the door for good. Usually though, a savvy clinical instructor will find those experienced nurses who have somehow avoided burnout, or haven't got there yet and will put students with them to learn from.

I entered nursing school not really knowing what I might want to do in the hospital, but I knew that there were many possibilities of what I might find interesting. I began clinicals in the various rotations at the hospitals my nursing school. Clinicals don't show you everything, but they show you enough. It was apparent with each one that these places were not for me. Med-Surg? No. With all of the various types of Med-Surg floors like pulmonary, GI, orthopedics, neuro, and others, they all had the same thing in common: burnt out nurses. Pediatrics? No. I could complete nursing tasks step by step, but didn't have the unique nurturing qualities that a nurse needs for children in the hospital. Critical care? The patient assignments were usually only one or two per nurse, but I wasn't so sure about seeing the same patients and families for weeks at a time, and then seeing some of them die. Emergency room? "IMA KILL ALL Y'ALL IF I DON'T GET MY DRUGS!" was all I needed to hear during one of my clinicals. Psych? No, and during that clinical in late junior year, I was beginning to wonder if I needed to be there myself because I still had not found what I wanted to do upon graduating. Mother/Baby and Labor and Delivery? NO. Good nurses in all of these places have qualities that suit them uniquely for their task. There were positive elements too in all of them but I still hadn't found my place yet and by senior year I was considering dropping out or switching majors.

I was on one of these units in my last year where I knew I didn't belong when there arose the need for my nurse preceptor and I to go down to the OR. I don't even remember why we had to go, but it was a chance to leave the unit so I was all for it. "A little field trip to kill some time and get this shift over with sooner" I thought to myself. What a terrible mindset, but that was where I was. The closer we came to the OR, the fewer people there were in the hallways. I felt as though I was being taken to a place hidden from view. Away from the waiting rooms, away from the visitors stopping you asking for directions, away from the large PR posters for the hospital hanging in every common area. Through a couple of badge-access doors and long hallways, we found ourselves at a desk station behind a wall of clear glass. A nurse sitting at the desk looked up at us. We were at "the board."

My preceptor began talking to the other nurse as I began reading the lines on the screens. I saw all of the procedures listed for that day, some I recognized, many I did not. I looked past the doors near the board and saw people passing by, everyone wearing either a tightly drawn surgical hat or puffy light blue one that looked like a hair net. Everyone there wore different scrubs than the floor nurses. A strip of red linoleum   on the floor separated where we stood and the hallway beyond. A sign on the wall said, "SURGICAL ATTIRE ONLY BEYOND THIS LINE."

The people walking on the other side of the red line glanced at us from behind their masks, seeing the strangers looking in from the edge of their world. I could tell even then that OR people had a way of communicating without saying a word. I felt suspicion, but also curiosity in their gazes as they quickly passed by us at the board. My own curiosity was growing with each minute we were there. Someone pushed an enormous machine down the hallway that made the floor vibrate as it passed by us. I asked what it was. "That's a microscope" said the OR nurse. This microscope was the size of a small car. I felt as though I was at the entrance of Willy Wonka's factory. After hearing numerous times from my teachers that the OR "wasn't real nursing," I felt rebellious just being there. It was soon time for us to return to the unit. I didn't want to leave. I wanted to know more.

That night I e-mailed my clinical instructor about getting into the OR for my last clinical in the spring semester. She replied that we could talk about it when I saw her next. My school was heavy on Med-Surg clinical visits, not so much for places like the OR. I had glimpsed a forbidden world, I wanted to return and explore. When I saw her later in the week, I was met with the same criticisms. "You'll lose your nursing skills in the OR...the patients aren't awake, and when they are, they don't remember you anyway...the surgeons are nasty...the nurses are nasty, THE OR ISN'T REAL NURSING."

My whole time in nursing school, we were told these things whenever the topic of surgery came up in a lecture and no more was ever said. When I actually saw for myself a brief look into this world, I knew right away there was more for me to find out. "Well, people really don't do the OR for their last clinical..." she kept on. I wasn't hearing it. With each passing clinical rotation, I was getting more convinced to leave nursing for good. For what?

I didn't know, but anything else had to be better. Finally, I had found something I wanted to know more about. My instructor finally relented and got me in touch with a preceptor in the OR. My journey behind the red line was about to begin!

Chapter 2. Or Nurses Are Real Nurses

At last! I had a clinical rotation I was looking forward to. Eight clinicals of eight hours each spread out over eight weeks. It was the first time I remember feeling real anticipation at an upcoming clinical in nursing school. I recall showing up to the OR excited that I would not have to wear my all-white nursing student scrubs all day. I had always hated wearing them so much. I used to wear boxers with bright stripes or darkly colored patterns that I knew would be seen through my thin white scrubs. A few of my friends in nursing school would always get a laugh as I walked up to them as we waited to begin whatever clinical we were on. Some days they saw stripes, some days they saw bright red hearts barely concealed by the cheap white cotton material. The longer I was in nursing school, the less I cared what my instructors thought of my see-through scrub bottoms. As I changed in the OR locker room into my light blue scrubs the hospital provided, I had no idea the things I would find out that had been misrepresented to me about the OR.

I was paired with a middle-aged nurse named Mike that immediately made me feel welcome on the unit. He took the time from the beginning to explain what made the OR different than other places in the hospital. Mike began his work day with a steady but calm approach, unlike the frenzy that seemed to always be present in other places I had been in the hospital. I would later find that sometimes the schedule demands of the OR can cause nurses to get stressed, but Mike was able to adapt his approach to the situation and still get the job done. He was the role model I needed to show me that it was possible to learn things about the OR other than what I had been told all through nursing school.

The first myth about the OR that I found wasn't true was the one that says your patients don't remember you. It's true that once you take them back into the OR, the sedatives and anesthesia medications take over. Without the advancements in anesthesia, most of today's surgeries couldn't take place. For this reason it is good that during the surgery, the patients don't remember you or anything about the OR. However, there are even many surgical procedures that use anesthetic methods called regional or local "blocks" where very specific areas of the body are made to lose feeling, and the patient stays either totally awake or slightly sedated and they are still able to converse with the members of the surgical team. So even though many patients are indeed asleep during surgery, there is a significant time before the surgery when you see your patient face to face.

Before the patient is brought back to the operating room, the surgical team meets with the patient in a place that most hospitals refer to as the holding room or pre-op. Most of the time a family member is also present with the patient before they are transported back into the operating room. While the patient is fully awake and before they have received any sedatives, the circulating nurse, the nurse anesthetist, anesthesiologist, and the surgeon all see the patient face to face and ask questions that are pertinent to each person's contribution to the patient's care. Of course, if an unconscious trauma patient arrives straight from the emergency room or if a patient is coming from a critical care unit, the surgical team will not be able to get answers from the patient directly. Other methods are used to confirm important safety measures before a patient is taken to surgery.

Unless the patient is unconscious as is usually the case if they are coming from the ICU, the patient is very much awake during this pre-op encounter. They haven't been allowed to eat since the night before, their normal clothes have been replaced with a big ugly gown that is open in the back, they have had IVs started in their arms or in other places on their body, and they are usually in pain of some kind, otherwise they would not be getting surgery! For many patients even if they have had surgery before, they are anxious and afraid because for all the knowledge and skills the surgeons have, they cannot promise they will leave the operating room with their problem completely taken care of. Surgeons try to anticipate every difficulty before beginning a surgery, but for very challenging procedures, the desired outcome is not always possible. This is especially true if the patient is already very ill to begin with. Receiving anesthesia also carries its own risk. These things and other factors can make patients very anxious.

Some surgeries, especially those that are cancer-related, can bring great stress into the patient's life. Imagine living your life normally with all of its mundane events but without the specter of cancer looming over you. One day you notice a lump somewhere that gets a little bigger each time you feel it or begin having terrible headaches accompanied with blurred vision. Things like that are unavoidable. You go to your regular doctor who refers you to a specialist. You are sent for costly x-rays and scans and after seeing the results, the doctor recommends surgery to retrieve some tissue to determine if it is cancer causing your symptoms. The day of surgery for these patients must be unimaginably stressful for them and their families. They may have several months of cancer treatment ahead of them or get the news that the cancer is already so insidious they only have months to live. Hopefully, the patient gets the news that the tissue causing their problems is benign and merely removing it will stop their symptoms.

Surgery and a hospital stay are very expensive, so many people can also be stressed about paying for their surgery. I have seen many times there will be a delay in the holding room because the patient's insurance company hasn't yet approved all or part of a patient's surgical plan. The same day they are there for surgery! As long as it is appropriate, the surgeon will sometimes either alter or change completely the procedure at the patient's request to make the cost of their care less burdensome. I have also seen a surgeon on the phone with an insurance company right before the patient is about to go into the OR explaining why the patient needs the treatment they need. How ridiculous!

Patients can also have worry about returning to their baseline abilities after a surgery, whether for work or leisure. Many people are the primary caregiver to older relatives or children and that is also something that can weigh on someone about to get surgery. How will the people they take care of be taken care while they recuperate from surgery? They may be wondering if their job is at risk if they cannot recover from their surgery. Sometimes people never return to their previous abilities before an injury, or a surgeon is not able to completely repair what was injured. The ideal result of any given surgery is to return the patient to their previous baseline; this is not always possible. The person's illness may too advanced to overcome, or the patient develops post-operative complications.

With all or some of these things running through a patient's head before surgery, it is the circulator's job and everyone else's on the surgical team to present a confident demeanor to the patient and their family. They may have already been waiting for a few hours for the surgical team to meet them, so they might already be impatient. The patient will be lying in a stretcher or hospital bed looking up at you in their vulnerable state. These beds are usually at waist-level to someone standing over them, so in their hungry, barely-clothed, painful existence, you must communicate assurance and calm to them. The patients need to know that with all of the stressors they are bringing with them to the operating room that day, wondering about the abilities of the surgical team aren't going to be one of them. So yes, the patient will remember you and the family will too, even if you only see them for a few minutes in the beginning of their time in the operating room. The surgeon will get more recognition and attention from the patient, but the nurse and others involved in their care are just as important.

In my pre-op "interview" or conversation with the patient, I stick to a prepared set of questions that may change depending on the type of surgery they are having. I begin my introducing myself and by explaining that I need to ask some specific questions about their surgery. I will discuss these questions more specifically in a later chapter. I try to find something I can banter with the patient about right before I begin my questions. I want to build some rapport with them even if just for a moment but also to replace the problems I've just written about and make them think about answers to my questions. Maybe the family member is wearing something with a sports team logo and I can comment on how well the team is playing or ask what they think about the new player the team just signed. Sports is a great conversation ice-breakers if you know what you're talking about and stay uncontroversial. Don't make the patient agitated with a reminder that their team just got beaten by a major rival! Perhaps the family is wearing a tourist shirt or hat that says where they visited and I can ask what it was like there or share my own experience from my visit if I had been there. I do keep things brief, usually under two minutes. It's plenty of time to find out what I need to know but also leave an impression.

Many hospitals already have or are starting to have policies that allow the OR staff to give surgical updates to the patient's families. Even after saying "see you later" (it's bad form to say "goodbye" to the family when rolling the patient's stretcher toward the OR), the nurse will call the patient's family in the waiting room to give an update. Usually, the nurse calls right after the first incision and every hour up until the end of surgery. For the family, waiting is the hardest part and a brief reassuring phone call can help their anxiety. The hospital may even have a screen that is displayed in the waiting room, with the patient's name and procedure removed to protect privacy. The family usually has the surgeon's name and a unique identifying number to watch on the screen as the surgery progresses. Most times the nurse will give a very generic update on the phone such as "we are still operating and I will give another update in an hour." Unless the surgeons themselves want to step to the phone to give a brief update, this is what usually happens. Oftentimes the surgery may be going well but the surgeon can't step away to talk on the phone. The families may want more specific information, but it would be very inappropriate for the nurse to comment to a family member on the phone on how well or how poorly a surgery is going. This is because the outcome of a surgery can change very quickly based on the surgeon's actions or on things out of the surgeon's control. Those conversations are best left to the surgeons to discuss with the family after surgery is over. If something dire occurs that wasn't expected during surgery and the family needs to be told, an OR nurse might need to ask whether an OR manager or the surgeon needs to speak to the family instead.

The idea that a nurse going into the OR will "lose their nursing skills" is one comment I've heard thrown around by nurses who have never been there. In fact, you develop other skills that nursing school and other units in the hospital have no capacity to teach you. If by nursing skills you mean starting IVs, giving NG tube feedings, and giving injections, then yes you could say a nurse could fall out of practice by not doing these things. However if a nurse goes back into a specialty where these tasks are common, you merely start doing them again and within a few weeks a good nurse adapts to their new reality. I haven't started an IV in years but I didn't forget how to! OR nurses still put in foley catheters and actually it's far easier in the OR because you don't put one in until the patient is asleep under anesthesia. The patient lies still and doesn't look at you while you're maneuvering a tube into their genitals. Sterility is easier to maintain as well because there aren't awake patients with dementia trying to kick you while you put a foley in. I never got added satisfaction putting in a foley because the circumstances were harder; make it as easy as possible!

A nursing skill you learn in nursing school and in practice on the floors is patient positioning and transferring them from one place to another. Specifically, this usually refers to moving them from their bed to a bedside toilet or from a wheelchair to their bed, etc. Hospitals can insist upon their staff using correct ergonomic practices and having two or three people at all times to help move a patient in their training videos and annual staff education, but nurses in the real world know this doesn't always happen. A nurse may not be able to wait for extra people to help move a patient because a confused patient with poor mobility has already gotten out of bed and is about to fall. The ideal situation isn't always reality and a nurse may have to step in alone to help them back to their bed. In the OR the patient is usually unconscious when you are moving them so they truly cannot contribute to their own movement. For this reason, it is an absolute necessity to have four or more people helping to move the patient. This team always includes the nurse anesthetist and the circulating nurse and may include other nurses and surgical staff. You simply cannot proceed with surgery until there are that many people helping to move the patient. There are numerous co-workers to enlist in helping you move a patient and the process of lifting and moving a patient is thankfully a shared effort. Often the surgeons and anesthesiologists themselves will help. The surgeons are very detail-oriented and want every limb exactly where they want them. The anesthesiologists and the nurse anesthetists want to make sure the patient's airway is protected and conducive to getting the oxygen they need during the case. So if you ask me: do I want the nursing skill where I hope I have enough help to move a patient and don't hurt my back in the process? Or do I want the nursing skill where I have multiple work peers invested in a good outcome that they are present next to me for every patient transfer? I know which one I want to have.

A necessary trait that is universal in nursing practice but is more profoundly used in the operating room is that of patient advocacy. In a hospital room the patient themselves are awake to give feedback on their care and often the family is there as well to offer their insight. In the operating room after the patient is asleep, their voice and their family's voice goes away and the nurse must step in to guard their interests. I think most patients don't even realize the great trust they are placing in the OR staff when they sign their consent forms. They have made a judgment whether or not to trust the surgeon with their care, and of course that is a significant decision. But the patient only meets the OR staff on the day of surgery, often only within a half hour of going off to sleep. Nearly every decision an OR nurse can make a good or bad outcome for a patient. Even something as simple as cleaning an operating room correctly makes the environment safer for the patient. An OR that is cleaned appropriately makes it less likely that a patient will acquire an infection. One that is not cleaned the right way can promote the spread of harmful microorganisms which can cause preventable harm.

Patient advocacy when practiced by the nurse in the OR can prevent serious mistakes from happening. For all their knowledge and experience that surgeons possess from their grueling education, they are still humans. They work long hours and almost every surgeon that operates in a main hospital has "call" of some kind. Call is what is known as the time when a nurse or doctor is expected to provide patient care outside of their normal working hours. If a surgeon is in a very busy specialty and there are few peers of their own to share the load, they may be called upon to operate all night. They still must provide their expertise even if they have normally scheduled operations the next day. Sometimes they may be able to postpone those other surgeries and rest a few hours, but not always. Scheduled time, or "block time" as it is called in the OR, is very valuable time set aside for surgeons to do their cases and most surgeons won't let it go unused if they can help it. During these times when a surgeon may be stretched thin on rest, the other members of the surgical team should be confident enough to speak up if they see something that was overlooked in the patient's care. Nurses might not be trained to understand things outside their scope of practice such as a surgeon's operating technique or clinical decision-making. Yet if a surgeon forgets to sign the patient's body part with their initials in pre-op, or they want to give an antibiotic that the patient is known to have a severe reaction to, then the nurse must step in and voice their concern. Indeed nurses and scrub techs take call too, but extra sets of eyes in the OR and the voices that go along with them are very important to keep patients safe.

Another misconception about nurses in the OR losing their skills is that they stop giving medications to patients. This is not true! The nurse anesthetists, or CRNAs do give many medications to the surgical patient through IVs during procedures. These drugs are used to provide anesthetic care, as well as pain relief. The CRNAs also have the priority responsibility of maintaining the patient's airway. Nurses however also deliver a wide variety of drugs to the patient, even if indirectly. For any given surgery a patient may need irrigating fluid with antibiotics added, local anesthetic with very specific concentrations and amounts, hemostatic agents (drugs that help to control bleeding), and other medications formulated for surgical use. A circulating nurse has to obtain the drugs the surgeon needs and check them against the patient's chart to make sure there will not be any harmful side effects. The nurse and the scrub tech must then prepare and label the medications clearly and correctly so that there is no confusion which container on the sterile table is holding what medication. Almost every medication that may be used in surgery is a clear liquid. With three or four medicine cups filled with various drugs it is obvious that special attention is needed to prevent confusion. Labels are handwritten and stuck to these cups and syringes to keep them from being misidentified. The surgeons are provided with the medications to give the patient and the nurse keeps track of how much was given so that the information can be added to the chart. Accurately charting medications is a necessity not only so that other healthcare professionals can see what was given, but also so that the patient is billed appropriately. Believe me, an OR nurse handles plenty of medications every single day.

One nursing task that is rarely done elsewhere in the hospital is dealing with tissue specimens. OR nurses have the very important task of retrieving tissue specimens from the surgical field, preparing and labeling them correctly, and sending them to the pathology lab where lab techs and pathologists analyze the specimens to determine what disease may be present. If a surgeon needs to know immediately what kind of cellular material is present, the nurse has to quickly prepare and send the specimen. This is especially important when handling cancerous tissue because the surgeon needs to determine if they have taken enough cancerous tissue out. For such a specimen, the nurse will open a sterile container and either the scrub person or surgeon will place the specimen inside. The nurse then must document and create a sticker label for the specimen, confirm the information is correct, and then call for a surgical team member to transport the specimen immediately to the hospital's pathology office. A pathologist will analyze the specimen and as soon as possible they will call the OR where the specimen came from and talk to the surgeon about what they see. This may determine whether or not the surgeon needs to remove more surrounding tissue. The types of cells the pathologist sees might also determine the type of treatment the surgeon chooses for the patient. This task may not sound all that challenging for the nurse, but when this process is done for multiple specimens in rapid succession, an OR nurse must stay organized and focused so that a mistake isn't made. Sending these specimens must be done quickly and correctly so that time is not wasted while the patient is lying on the operating table. Specimens can be as small as tiny biopsy portions you can barely see or entire sections of colon that weigh five pounds or more. Other types of specimens may not need to be sent urgently, but they still must be collected and documented correctly. If a specimen isn't being sent to pathology right away, or if no time-sensitive analysis is needed, a specimen may be placed in a container with a liquid preservative called formalin. The nurse has to be careful not to touch the formalin because it can cause burns to the skin. OR nurses have this unique task because a surgeon cannot step away to handle and transport specimens, and other staff members scrubbed into a case have their own responsibilities.

The nursing responsibility of delegation also is something OR nurses are not left out of. A floor nurse has many people to delegate tasks to: a CNA, cleaning staff, unit secretary, other nurses, and hospital transport staff. I'm sure I left some others out, but the idea of delegation is enlisting the skills of other hospital staff to perform tasks specific to their roles so that the nurse can focus on nursing tasks. Cleaning a spill in a patient's room is important, but it is more appropriate to have a cleaning staff person perform that role while a nurse does things only a nurse can do. If an OR nurse tried to perform every single task that happens behind the scenes before a patient is brought back for surgery, there would be an hour gap (at best!) between each case. In most surgical departments, there are additional staff to help transport patients to pre-op, assist nurses and surgeons to position patients, clean rooms after cases, and get equipment ready for future cases. There are many other tasks these staff may do, but these are the major ones that OR nurses cannot do without. An OR nurse has to recognize when there are things best left to other people so that they can focus on doing patient specific assessments and tasks. Delegating at its best occurs when there is a teamwork mindset; at its worst, a poor nurse lets laziness or bossy-ness set the tone and it drags down everyone around them.

Having great people skills is a universal workplace trait that everyone knows is beneficial. I will explain here the importance it plays in the operating room specifically.

Nurses need to build rapport with other nurses and surgeons because it makes it easier to speak up and express concerns when they arise. Ideally, all surgeons are also open to building good work relationships with the people they spend hours at a time with every day. This isn't always the case, and just like nurse have their favorite surgeons to work with, surgeons also have their favorite scrub techs and nurses. New OR nurses can often have difficulty starting these relationships; indeed this is one of the most common barriers new people face when first starting in the OR. People already in the OR have established relationships and backgrounds with each other based upon long hours working together and shared experiences. It doesn't take long for a new person to hear "war stories" from old-timers. Nevertheless, an OR nurse has to cultivate at minimum some communication skills that allow them to speak up with confidence if they see something being done incorrectly or unsafely, even if the surgeon they are with is unfamiliar to them or seems unapproachable. This can be difficult to do; unfortunately OR culture as a whole in the past has been very favored toward the surgeon's authority and any questioning by others is seen as being insubordinate or "difficult." Without a doubt surgeons have great knowledge, but some are very capable of cutting corners and letting their egos cause mistakes.

A new nurse in the OR will soon pick up on different ways to communicate other than speaking. Reading the temperature of an OR if you're walking in to give someone a break or give a permanent relief is very important. If I'm going into a surgery I didn't have a part in getting started, I always take a few seconds to look at people's body language through the door or window of an OR so I at least try to get a feel for what I'm walking into. Ideally, everyone in the room is calmly performing their roles. Circumstances may make a surgery stressful, so it's wise to know this and adjust accordingly so the stress isn't amplified by loudly talking to someone in the corner of the room. Since our faces are covered by masks, we in the OR get good at making others know what we need just through eye contact. It isn't always wise to shout across the room during a tense or challenging portion of a surgery. The surgeon may be encountering a very difficult or unexpected event during the case and any loud distraction could result in an error along with a searing glare from the surgeon in your direction, with or without some words. A scrub can intimate and point with their eyes to what they need without yelling in the surgeon's ear they're standing right next to. Building rapport by working with the same people all the time fosters this type of communication.

Communication is also key in the OR because nurses talk to pre-op and PACU (post-anesthesia care unit) nurses every day and people in many other places in the hospital, and thus need to have a good working relationship with them. I call the hospital pharmacy and blood bank often, and I speak to the family waiting room volunteers and answer pages from the surgeon's beepers and phones every single shift I work. There are also people called "reps," or representatives that are allowed in the OR to guide the surgeons using their company's medical devices and/or implants. Sometimes these reps have a medical background, but these are usually people with sales and business experience that are trained by their companies to know every detail about their products and answer any questions and troubleshoot issues that might arise during a surgery. A nurse or surgeon using a new piece of equipment or set of surgical instruments relies heavily on their guidance and it's always beneficial to have a good working relationship with them.

Speaking of equipment and instruments just now, let me also describe something that is also special about the OR. Nurses and scrub techs in the OR do more than just hand the surgeon instruments when they ask for something. Beyond just knowing the names of the thousands of instruments and products available to use in the OR, the staff has to know what the instrument they're holding is, what it's used for, and whether or not it's in proper working order. A new nurse to the OR slowly builds their knowledge about the vast number of instruments they might see, but looking at a table full of instruments laid out on an OR table can be overwhelming and intimidates many good nurses just starting out. Seasoned OR nurses know it takes time for new people to learn instruments, so beginners are usually started out learning a few dozen instruments that are used for a wide variety of surgeries. As months go by for a new person, they remember the instruments they see every day and learn new ones as they continue on. A nurse that works mainly in one specialty becomes very familiar with the unique instruments for their types of surgeries. An ortho nurse is more comfortable wielding power drills and saw blades than a general surgery nurse for example. Safely using and passing instruments to another surgical team member is also crucial; a careless or ignorant nurse can injure themselves or someone else if they do not handle the instruments correctly. Many instruments have sharp pieces or moving parts that can easily pass through surgical gloves and cause injuries.

All of these things about the OR I've just described are things I never knew from the outside looking in until I actually made it there in my nursing school clinical and eventually as a full-time nurse. "Anyone can do the OR" is an insult I heard from people in nursing school. The implication was that working in the OR was for people who couldn't make it elsewhere in the hospital and it wasn't anything special. I think any nurse would agree by now that this isn't so, even if they don't like what they already know about the OR. Likewise, an OR nurse couldn't be expected to go to another unit and pick up where they left off in nursing school clinicals on a standard med-surg unit. I am grateful I had the chance to have a dedicated clinical to the OR in nursing school. It led me into a challenging, but interesting career.

My OR nursing school clinical was over before I knew it, and I left wanting more. I was hooked! I was fascinated by all the instruments and the skill the surgeons and nurses had. I saw things right in front of me I had only read about in my text books. The diseases and injuries that caused so much pain in the patients I saw weekly in the hospital were being actively treated by surgical teams that impressed me more and more the longer I saw them work. Most of the patients that came to the hospital I saw were suffering from their symptoms of their illnesses; I saw in the OR active solutions being carried out to alleviate that suffering. Surgery alone cannot end all the pain someone might have, and there are side effects of surgery itself to manage, but it was this idea that solidified my desire to know more about the OR. I spent the last weeks of nursing school wearing a wry grin when I was with my classmates, feeling I knew secrets they didn't. Many of them had also found their niche and probably felt the same way. After graduation, the stressful time of job applications and studying for and taking the NCLEX began.

You might be expecting now to hear that I found my first OR job in an exciting city and began working only months after nursing school as I found the joyful purpose in my life as an OR nurse, all before turning 23. Such a storyline would perfectly end this chapter and I could begin the next one talking about the things about the workplace culture in the OR that inspired me to begin writing this book in the first place. This however is not the case.

Chapter 3. Making It In

When I graduated more than ten years ago, getting a foothold in the OR was more difficult than it is today. Even now it is still somewhat more challenging to get that first chance compared to other places in the hospital. Large hospitals either would only hire experienced nurses, meaning nurses from other areas in the hospital or OR nurses from other hospitals. If some hospitals had training programs for OR nurses, again they would either only accept experienced nurses or they would only offer them as demand for more staff arose within the OR. One hospital from my hometown I applied to chose not to offer their OR training program the summer I graduated because there weren't enough open positions in their OR to fill. I grew crestfallen as I found that the hospitals I wanted to work for had the same stipulations in their job listings for OR nurses: "one year nursing experience required," "OR experience required," "prior OR experience a must." I had heard that getting into the OR could be difficult; my desire to be an OR nurse would overcome any trouble I had in landing a position I told myself.

In hindsight, if I had expanded the locations where I could have found a new nurse program into the OR, I probably could have found one. Doing so might have meant moving a few states away from family and this was something I refused to do. Looking back, I know I could have done it. It would have been easy to move; I had not married yet and didn't have kids. At the time I didn't understand that trying to follow a dream might mean making some sacrifices. After all, it didn't have to be permanent.

Instead of potentially finding my way into the OR from day one, I chose to follow the path that seemingly was the only one for me to take: work as a floor nurse for the minimum one year and then begin applying to the OR. Truthfully, a nurse with experience elsewhere in the hospital does have a clear advantage over someone with no work experience. Experienced nurses in general usually have good troubleshooting skills and having to critically think through problems is a skill you have to have working in the hospital. As I've already said, a nursing student just doesn't have this yet. It's possible for a newly graduated nurse to start and thrive in the OR, but it's rare.

I began working as a night shift Med-Surg nurse for a Neuro unit at one of the main hospitals where I lived. My shift was three 12 hour shifts each week. I made slightly more money working on nights rather than days, but it was one of the least favorite jobs I've ever had. Not only was it not the job I wanted, the schedule itself beat me up. I was a terrible sleeper in the daytime and usually only could sleep four or five hours max on my days off. Black out shades, earplugs, and eye covers couldn't overcome my body telling itself "this isn't normal, why are you doing this to yourself?" When I had two or more days off between work days, I couldn't simply re-adjust and sleep at night. I would be groggy all day, and then be wide awake from 8 in the evening until about 3 in the morning. My eyes were always bloodshot. When I worked, I would drive home half asleep after a night shift, with the blinding light of the sunrise in my eyes the entire way home. People on their way to work in the cars around me had just had a normal night's sleep; I often felt on the verge of nodding off just long enough to swerve off the road. In the evening as people in my neighborhood were grilling in their back yards and settling in after their work day, I was off again to work. The sunset mocked me through my windshield that I was about to work for twelve hours and drag myself back home somehow in the morning.

After a few months of little sleep combined with the grueling work load of standing and walking for most of my shift, I developed chronic back pain and began going to see a chiropractor. I was in my early 20's and in decent physical shape, how could this be happening?! I even bought a pair of orthopedic shoes from the shoe aisle reserved for elderly mall walkers. I absolutely hated it. Some people thrive working night shift; I was not one of them.

The work was everything I expected from nursing school, except that no one tells you about the feeling of not having enough time to do your work. I had 5 or 6 patients every shift. Some of the patients were very easy to care for and were mostly self-sufficient, but some of them were so ill I found myself looking in on them every half hour to assess for changes in their status. Some people were so sick I was in their rooms for one reason or another the majority of my shift, all the while worried that I was missing someone else's needs in another room. I struggled to do my charting correctly and in time whenever I was out of the room and also do other nursing responsibilities whenever I wasn't taking care of a patient. In the first six months, I often felt as I walked out my car at the end of my shift that I had neglected the other patients in my care. If there were other needs to be met that I knew about, I would call my charge nurse to see my other patients temporarily. I hated the feeling of being stretched too thin.

Even with a CNA and a charge nurse to rely on, 6 patients can be very challenging for one nurse. The floor was a stark contrast to the OR where a whole surgical team had one patient at a time and everyone could concentrate on their responsibility. Many people with Med-Surg experience that switch to the OR did so for this reason I've learned from conversations with peers. I kept working hard with the memory of my nursing school OR rotation in my mind. Around the six month mark I felt more confident in my abilities to manage my time as a floor nurse, but the desire for the OR remained.

Before long my year anniversary had passed and I began applying to OR positions in my area. The hospital I was in had open positions, so I applied. I also looked at other places around me to apply to; by now I was more than willing to jump to another hospital if it meant getting off the floor and into my desired workplace. A major nationally-recognized teaching hospital in the area had a OR training program I applied to. In a few weeks I was scheduled for an interview and I excitedly anticipated my chance.

I arrived there and was shown to a waiting room with a few other people. My scheduled time was for 1:00, but didn't get called in to start until about 1:30. As I walked into the room and was introduced to the team of three people conducting the interview, someone brought in two large bags of Chinese takeout. One interviewer was visibly irritated at me as I approached her to shake her hand; I had kept her from her egg roll for an extra five seconds. This interview was off to a bad start.

I sat down and the main interviewer offered a quick apology that they were about to eat and not to let it distract me from the interview. No problem, I thought. As I sat there, my heart pounding as I waited for the first question, all three of them hurriedly opened their food and began squirting soy sauce and duck sauce on their plates...and began eating...and not talking. After a few minutes, I filled the silence by asking if everyone had a copy of my resume(they didn't), and when the training program would start(they would discuss it). Eventually, the main person sitting in the middle picked up a piece of paper and slid her takeout box to the side. She said nonchalantly, "well we already have several people from this morning we think we're probably going with, but let's see what you've got." I could feel the look on my face sink, but I said something to the effect of "ok, let's do it." I stood to hand out three copies of my resume to the three nurses in front of me. The two interviewers on both sides barely looked at it, and neither of them would pick up a pen during my interview. The middle person quickly glanced at it and began jotting down quick notes as her questions began. I was irritated with each passing question because it was obvious two of the people weren't listening as I watched fried rice fall off their forks as they ate, and the main interviewer was hurrying along the list of questions to get on to the next person. The interview was over in less than ten minutes, and I left knowing my pitch to get a spot in the program wasn't enough. I've heard of people giving tough interviews to see how the candidate will react. This situation didn't feel like that. Looking back, I feel certain they had already found who they wanted and were trying to get finished with interviews for the day.

As I drove on the interstate back home, I was crestfallen. Were all of my OR interviews going to be like that? My Med-Surg interview went just as quick, but I left knowing I would be offered the job because the floor was so short-staffed. I pulled off the highway and ate at a restaurant. As I sat eating my own late lunch, I stewed on the joke of an interview I had just left. I was annoyed at the unprofessionalism and thought less of the organization who prided themselves on the headlines their hospital generated. I resolved to keep applying though; I had my work experience now and deeper knowledge of the OR that many applicants probably didn't have. I sped back onto the interstate as I headed home and I tried my best to put the last few hours in the past. Ironically, years later I would find myself on the other side of the interview table at that same hospital interviewing candidates to be in the same training program. I became a nurse educator there and by the time I had arrived, the people that had brushed me off in my interview weren't there anymore. More about that chapter in my life is yet to come.

A few weeks after the Chinese food interview, a friend told me about the OR training program she had just finished at another hospital in another nearby city. I still had not heard anything from the OR at my current hospital and my hope was fading of leaving the floor. I applied to my friend's hospital and soon had another interview scheduled. I don't remember the time of day I went, but I'm pretty sure it was the earliest one available! Again I wore my best interview outfit and splashed Visine in my eyes before walking in (I still had the night shift look going on!). When I walked in, none of the interviewers had trays of food in front of the them, so I felt I was already improving my chances of having a better interview. Introductions were had and we all sat down to begin. There were two upper level directors of the OR and the main educator who ran the OR training program. I briefly discussed my resume, but spent far more time talking about the experience from my nursing school OR clinical and the profound impact it made on me. I absolutely name-dropped my friend who had just been through the program, as I was certain she was a good worker and was getting along well in the OR. I asked many questions about the program itself and the expectations they had from people in the program. After about a half hour, I left with far more confidence of my chances of getting called back. I even left for work that night hopeful that my night shifts would soon be coming to an end.

I spent the next week exhausted from work like normal, checking my e-mail for new messages and keeping my phone close to catch any phone calls telling me some good news. I think I even kept the ringer on my phone turned up as I slept after work so I wouldn't miss any potential good news. Sure enough, about two weeks later I got word that they wanted me to start the training program in 6 weeks. I was ecstatic! This was it! I waited about one week at work before I gave my month notice. My manager was disappointed, but they were used to people leaving. It seemed like someone was leaving every other month from my unit. Even with new people starting occasionally, we had a hard time staying fully-staffed. Someone told me when they heard the news I wouldn't feel like I had any more free time when I started working day shift. I laughed out loud and said thanks for the warning. I couldn't wait to be back on days, even if it meant five days a week. Whatever "extra" time night shift people had came at a cost, and I was over paying for it.

For me, making it into the OR took persistence, showing the interviewers that I already had an idea what the

OR was like, and having people in the OR I knew that I could ask questions and keep me informed of openings. The persistence was necessary since I had to be willing to put in the nursing work experience, even if it wasn't where I wanted to be in the beginning. There was also the waiting and applying for openings that didn't happen in a matter of a week. The OR clinical in nursing school I did was something I used to my benefit during the interview that landed me the starting position. If you are in nursing school and get even one day in the OR and find that you like it, try to get back there again for clinicals or see if the OR managers will let you come back to shadow. This is also something you can bring up in an interview if you apply for that same OR later if you did a clinical or shadow visit there. Take everything you learn about the OR from that brief time to make them understand you have at least been in the OR longer than a brief visit. Some people have preconceived notions about the OR when they apply and have never really seen what it's like. To an interviewer, someone who doesn't really know about the OR is easy to spot. They may have a sincere interest, but nurses with unrealistic expectations usually aren't selected into a training program and interviewers try to find this out. Finally, the handful of people I knew from nursing school and in the OR where I applied helped me know when to apply. The interviewers where I was accepted asked how I found out about the position and I told them about the person I knew from the last training program. They immediately nodded in approval when I told them who it was and I had zero hesitation using my association with them to my benefit. Networking is how lots of people get positions in many fields and any advantage you have should be used. The OR is no different.

I never heard any word from the OR position at my original hospital I had first applied for. Maybe the demand for new people fell or they filled it and didn't bother contacting me. It didn't matter, I had a new destination in front of me. I took a week off in between my last day on the floor and the first day of my training program. I made myself stay awake for the mornings in my week off and exercised in the afternoons. By the end of the week, I was going to sleep at 10 pm and it felt amazing to sleep seven or eight hours in a row. My back quit hurting as much. I really underestimated how important having a normal schedule was *for me.* There are people who can handle night shift like champs. It's certainly necessary to have people at all hours in the hospital for obvious reasons. I'm glad those special people exist. Most hospitals have full time night shift staff if the demand is there, and if not the day shift people take call. By and large though, if you work day shift in the OR you rarely work late into the evening or overnight consecutively, unless you've chosen such a schedule or picked up other nurse's call responsibilities. I was ready to put the night owl routine in the past and restart a normal working schedule.

Chapter 4. Training

I eagerly drove to my first day of the training program feeling well-rested and energetic. It was still nursing, but I felt as if I was starting a brand new career. I walked into the hospital that first morning with the multitudes of other nurses and hospital staff coming to work. Everyone's role could be identified by their scrub color, which differs from hospital to hospital. My polo shirt and khakis were a welcome contrast to me as I found my way to the hallway full of meeting rooms where we had been told to meet. I entered the room and met two other people also in the program. As three more people came in later and we introduced ourselves, it was obvious we all shared the same excitement of taking the first steps of making it into the OR.

The leader of the program arrived and began telling us what our next six months would look like. She told us our first month would be concentrated on lessons and practicing skills unique to the OR environment. We would then start clinicals in the main OR with dedicated preceptors for three or four weeks at a time in differing specialties. We were told to treat our clinicals like a working job interview because we would meet with the coordinators and managers from the OR to discuss the specialty openings. At the end of the program, we would be presented with the available specialty openings and choose our starting points in the OR. The hospital system I was now in had a main hospital that had been open since the early 1900's and in recent years had either built smaller hospitals in nearby communities or acquired ownership of other ones. We were told that while the main hospital would have the majority of openings, there were also opportunities in the OR at some of the other campuses.

We were each given a three ring binder with lecture materials and a schedule for the next six months. Before we knew it, the first day was over and we were dismissed for the day. I was really happy driving home in the middle of the afternoon; it felt like leaving school early! I don't know what I did the rest of that day, but it probably involved a run in my neighborhood or taking care of a necessary chore around the house. I was starting to experience the coveted "work-life balance" that I never felt I really had for the past year and a half.

The material in our training lessons was familiar to us already due to our nursing experience(no one in my group was fresh out of nursing school), but it was exciting because we were learning and practicing concepts related to the OR that weren't covered in nursing school. We learned about the room itself and how even the airflow inside a properly running operating room was meant to reduce the chance of spreading microorganisms to the patient. We practiced putting on surgical gowns and gloves correctly so that we could safely handle sterile surgical instruments. We heard from many OR nurses themselves as they visited us for a half hour or more to show us a piece of equipment or instrument tray that they used often in their specialty. With each passing day in that starting month I realized how much I had yet to learn about the OR, but this did not discourage me. In my nursing school OR clinical, I didn't always know the questions to ask about something I didn't understand. Now, I was feeling more equipped to ask questions and learn more.

My first week of not having any lectures or skill practice was spent in the sterile processing area of the main hospital. This is where all the surgical instruments are cleaned, repackaged, and sterilized before being used in another surgery. This was the ideal place to start because while it wasn't technically in the OR, I could spend time handling instruments and learning the names of about one hundred common ones that most every service used frequently. It was also beneficial to see what happens behind the scenes where the instruments are being prepared. There were twenty operating rooms at the main hospital and if one can imagine an average of three cases per room per day, with anywhere from two to 10 or more instrument trays per case, there would be a few hundred trays to clean, reorganize, package, sterilize, and store every day. I soon developed a big appreciation for what the sterile processing staff were able to accomplish. Later when I would work as a circulator and encounter a shortage in the supply room of a certain instrument tray I needed or if I found something wasn't cleaned properly, I would try to remember the volume of work they had to do and patiently ask someone to help me get what I needed rather than get frustrated.

The sterile processing workers put me and another of my peers to work cleaning dirty instruments and showing us the process of how we were able to correctly and safely reuse the surgical instruments. A used tray would arrive at one side of the department in an enclosed area where the first cleaning would take place. There was a long, deep metal sink where we sprayed and scrubbed the instruments until any visible contaminants were removed. Then the trays were placed in a large metal frame and rolled into a large washing machine that mostly resembled a large dishwasher. The instruments would pass out of the washer on the other side after the cycle into another separate room where the "clean" instruments would then be re-assembled neatly into their metal trays. After enclosing the trays, they were then placed along with several others onto a long metal rack where they would be moved into a large steam sterilizer. After sterilization was over and the trays had cooled for a few hours, they were sent to the supply room in the OR where nurses could get them straight off the shelf and take them into a case. There were a few instruments that could not be steam sterilized and required different types of decontamination and sterilization. I spent a day cleaning instruments, but spent the rest of the week reassembling instruments with an experienced worker and slowly learned the names of each one as I placed them neatly into their trays. By the end of the week, I had a good starting grasp on the main instruments.

After that week in sterile processing, we began our rotations through the various services picked out for us. I would spend two to three weeks on the General, Ortho, and Neuro teams as well as visit some of the other satellite hospitals in the system briefly.

My first team was General. There were about a dozen nurses and scrub techs who mainly did nothing but "general" cases. Without compiling a long list, these cases usually involved any illnesses with the GI tract or soft tissue. Many cancer cases were handled by the general team. The general surgeons would also be involved if a trauma surgery needed their help to repair or remove damaged organs.

I was paired with a veteran nurse who had been on the general team for several years. The first few days went well, I was picking up easy things and my preceptor and the other team members were introducing me to new things as I would show my ability to handle them. It was a good start because I told the team I had just started the program recently and they were my first rotation visit. They knew my OR skills were limited so they gave me appropriate things to test me. To any new nurse in the OR, I definitely suggest being up front with the people you meet so that they understand your experience level and can adjust their expectations of your work. The OR, like everywhere in the hospital, is no place to bluff or overstate your abilities.

Things were going great that first week. I was really in the OR and taking care of real patients alongside a great team. One morning later in the week, I met my preceptor at the assignment board and heard her say, "oh great" as she looked at our room number. The surgeon's name on the screen made someone else pass by and say "good luck!" My preceptor started her brisk pace toward our room and started talking. "Dr. Chen is good, but he really doesn't take to new people. I'll handle the big tasks today and you keep doing your thing." I shrugged and said ok and kept walking. I had heard surgeons could have tempers and not always be great to work with. It wasn't anything I was totally unfamiliar with; other doctors I had worked with had times they were impatient. As we came into the room, we began the first case routine of starting up the room equipment and opening the sterile supplies and instruments.

My preceptor drove the pace of getting started that morning. She already had the responsibility of training me, a new person, and working with a surgeon whose reputation apparently preceded him, I could tell she was a little more stressed than usual. We hurriedly got the room ready and were soon on the way to meet the patient and CRNA in the pre-op area. Our first case was a patient having their gallbladder removed laparoscopically. In a nutshell, the patient would have a few small incisions placed at various spots on their abdomen, their abdominal cavity would be inflated with CO_2, and narrow instruments and a lighted camera would be placed inside the body to find and remove the gallbladder. We talked to the patient and saw that everything with the chart was ready to go.

We set off toward our OR ahead of schedule. We entered the room five minutes before the time the managers wanted first cases to roll into their rooms. Everything was going great! The anesthesiologist came in almost right behind us and after we helped the patient move over onto the operating table, they were off to sleep. All of our beginning tasks were being checked off one by one. I could see my preceptor began to relax little by little; we were off to a smooth start. Counts were done, meds were given, the patient was asleep and positioned, and we had beat the clock. Nothing can derail a work day in the OR like a late start or some obstacle that will irritate the surgeon.

My preceptor and another nurse went over to the computer desk to call Dr. Chen to come to the room. I had been starting to "prep" the patients the day before; this is when the patient's skin is exposed where the incision will be and various cleaning products are used to greatly reduce or eliminate all of the microorganisms on the skin's surface. Because a surgical incision breaks the most important barrier the human body has to the outside world, the skin has to be completely clean and ready to handle the intrusion from the outside. My preceptor watched me put on sterile gloves, something else I was still getting the hang of. OR nurses have to put on sterile gloves in a certain way so that none of their skin touches the outside of the gloves. I put them on right the first time, another achievement in our morning! The scrub even said good job as they handed me the prep applicator. As I spread the bright orange cleaning liquid over the patient's abdomen, the nurses in the corner cracked a joke. The room had a laugh; "we've got this" was the general mood.

Dr. Chen walked into the room. He casually sauntered over to the desk and said a flat "good morning" to the other nurses. I was about to finish my prep and step away to hit the timer on the wall; the cleaning solution needed to air dry for three minutes due to the presence of alcohol in it. Dr. Chen walked over to me, and as I was about to introduce myself, he shouted, "WHAT ARE YOU DOING?! YOU'RE GOING TO GIVE MY PATIENT AN INFECTION!" I immediately looked in horror at my preceptor, whose face although half covered with a mask looked completely frozen. The rant was only beginning. "YOU LEFT THIS NASTY DIRT ALL OVER THE STOMACH, WHAT'S WRONG WITH YOU?!" I couldn't say anything, I didn't know what to say. I think I eventually managed to croak "what was I supposed to do?"

I kept looking at the nurses in the corner to do something, anything. I was getting torched. The bright OR lights above us in the middle of the room only amplified the dressing down. The CRNA fiddled with an IV that was completely fine; the scrub tech closely examined an instrument that she had been handling already the past ten minutes. Finally, the other nurse who wasn't even my preceptor walked over and asked Dr. Chen what he saw. He finally turned away from me and angrily pointed to some bits of sticky residue left by EKG pads on the side of the abdomen. "I'VE TOLD YOU PEOPLE NOT TO LEAVE THIS CRAP ON THE SKIN WHEN YOU'RE PREPPING!" The other nurse immediately went to the cabinet to get something. "I've got adhesive remover," she said as she rushed back to me. Dr. Chen turned away and stormed out of the room. I had just been initiated into the OR.

Slowly my preceptor finally said, "I wish I had seen you prepping, if there is sticker residue from the EKG pads the prep itself won't take it off." I thought to myself I could have really used that intervention when my face was melting off 30 seconds earlier, but as I looked down at my inadequate prepping, sure enough I could see the dark fuzzy mess still attached to the patient's skin beneath the orange colored film. My heart was racing; I thought I had done something truly unsafe and the patient was hurt. In hindsight, it was nothing. All we had to do was swipe the area a few times with the adhesive remover and re-prep. An extra few minutes. At the time, I simply didn't know it was an easy fix.

Dr. Chen re-entered the room a few minutes later. He silently re-inspected the prep and we continued with the procedure. I was no longer confident in myself but kept doing the things I knew to do. I would find that whoever the team was that worked with him was usually on egg-shells all or part of the day. My preceptor didn't really talk about the incident or how it unfolded. That's just how it was. A few hours later on my morning break, I went into the staff lounge. Taped to the door was a simple but unambiguous piece of paper that said in large font something like:

"All Staff, for all of Dr. Chen's cases from now on, please be sure that the surgical area is completely clear of any dirt or sticky residue before prepping!!"

My shock turned to anger. I found out that Dr. Chen had thrown a fit to the OR manager after storming out of our room and the response had been to print these sheets and tape them to the staff lounge doors as well as the locker room doors. My prepping disaster was hot gossip in the OR for the rest of the week. Luckily, whoever heard about it and asked me what happened responded with sympathy and encouragement that I wasn't the first person to have my head bitten off by Dr. Chen. I was really pissed though that the reaction was to make such a minor thing public, and no one in authority ever came to me, the new person to explain the situation.

Did the surgeon overreact? Yes. Did the preceptor let me get scorched? Yes. Did I ever forget to check a patient's abdomen for residue after that? Never. Could the situation have been handled in a more constructive way? Definitely. Did management make a knee-jerk decision and turn a potential teaching moment into an embarrassment? Yes.

Any feeling of teamwork I had with my preceptor vanished the rest of the time I was in general. I didn't trust her as much and I think she was irritated to have been associated with me during the surgeon's freak out. She taught me about general surgery but the incident also taught me to keep my head on a swivel in the OR. I wish the lesson had been less caustic, although I've never forgotten it.

I moved onto the Ortho team next. My reputation as a

lazy skin prepper followed me as I introduced myself to a new surgical team. It was encouraging to be met with off color jokes about Dr. Chen by the ortho nurses; if they ever had to be pulled to do a general case he was just as much of a jerk to them too they said. The ortho team handled any bone or joint disorders and also traumas. I was put with another experienced preceptor that quickly showed me many things I already knew but were more specific to orthopedics. The instruments in ortho were a huge change from general; there were huge drills and sharp drill bits, and hammers and chisels of all sizes. There were a lot fewer sharp instruments in general surgery besides the scalpel because anything sharp could puncture the bowel or other soft tissue. It seemed every instrument in the ortho trays were meant to cut, chisel, or drill.

I soon developed a great interest in ortho. The surgeries were very physical. There was lots of banging and sawing with bits of bone and blood flying in all directions from the surgical field. My preceptor quickly taught me when it was a good time to make our phone calls to patient's families in the waiting room for updates. We wanted to call when it didn't sound like a busy auto garage in the background. Clanging metal and loud drills would probably be very easy to hear over a phone since even if you were standing next to someone, you had to raise your voice to be heard during the noise.

The surgeons I encountered in ortho were intense but they recognized I was new and many took the time to quickly explain their surgeries as they were performing them. Many of them also had PAs, or physician assistants who came with them to the OR. The PAs usually stayed behind near the end of a case to close the incision and place dressings and casts while the surgeon would leave the OR to get a head start on getting ready for the next case. All the PAs I met were very friendly and would answer questions about the case that had just occurred.

I also was introduced to a special group of people in the OR with no medical licenses but are important to the team in many ways. In ortho, there was almost always an entourage around of ridiculously good-looking men and women wearing red surgical caps known as "reps." Seriously, almost all of them looked like they had stepped out of an Instagram account with half a million followers. Many of them were tanned and muscular and they all wore scrub sizes that were tight fitting, especially the women. Once before a case started, a certain rep wasn't in the room yet and the staff were trying to locate him. The hospital had just remodeled the main floor of the hospital which included almost an entire hallway of mirrors on both sides. The surgeon quipped, "check the main floor, he's probably looking at himself in the new mirrors."

The reps were polite to the staff, but we were not the main targets of their attention. They made sure everything the surgeon wanted was available. They always seemed to know when the surgeon had returned from a vacation or the condition of their child who had just suffered a sports injury. One time I saw a rep outside an OR hurriedly thumbing up the screen of his smart phone. As I was about to go in, the rep caught me and asked, "Are you friends with Dr. Adams on Facebook?" I said no and went about my business as he turned his face back to the phone. I later found out he was a newer rep to the surgical group and he was trying to "friend" all of the surgeons to get up to speed on their social media presence. He was trying to find someone's Facebook who already had that doctor "friended" before he walked into the room.

If it sounds like I'm criticizing, I'm not. While I was in the ortho rotation, I gained an appreciation for the reps in those cases and the value they brought to the patient's care. There were many ortho cases that needed eight or more trays just for implants and implant instruments. These trays could contain several hundred pieces in total and the reps knew the contents front to back and side to side. Instead of a scrub or nurse at the sterile table picking through each tray on their own, a rep would stand nearby and tell them exactly where to find a certain piece, assemble it, and make it ready to pass to the surgeon. The surgeons knew what the instruments and implants were for, but during a surgery their focus is on controlling bleeding and accessing the areas in the body that need to be repaired, they simply don't have time to look away to put instruments together. After scrubbing some cases in ortho, I was always appreciative of the rep's patience and help during the case.

All too soon my time in ortho was over, it had been a big improvement over my prior rotation. I was fascinated by the instruments and special tables that were used for all the types of surgeries I saw. I hoped at the end of my training I would be able to land a spot on the Ortho team. Unfortunately, there weren't any openings on their team but I was told things could change by the end of the training program.

I next went to the Neuro team. I was already interested in Neuro because that was where I had been in Med-Surg. Many of the floor patients I took care of were post-operative back surgeries or craniotomies. I was about to see how those surgeries took place. The Neuro team I met was very close-knit because there were fewer neurosurgeons compared to the number of surgeons in other specialties, so there weren't as many dedicated staff to neuro procedures.

I soon saw that many of the spinal procedures weren't as intriguing as some of the other surgeries you could see in the OR. The incision usually wasn't very big, and unless you were standing right over the patient, you couldn't see inside the body to see where the surgeon was working. The work was understandably steady and methodical. The surgeons were working around the patient's spinal cord when operating on the patient's back, and if they were operating on the patient's neck, they also had to be conscious of the patient's esophagus. I wasn't bored watching these surgeries, but the steps in each procedure were easy to follow because they were so repetitive.

My interest really grew with Neuro when I saw my first craniotomy. One day a patient was having a tumor removed and the coordinator placed me and my preceptor in the case. Every week so far in my training had shown me something that amazed me, and this would be no different. The patient was first brought in and helped to the operating table like always. After anesthesia was induced and the airway was secure, the surgeon came in and placed a metal headpiece around the patient's head with three sharp pins holding the frame in place on the patient's skull. The surgeon had looked at the patient's MRI and knew exactly where to place the headpiece so that he could position the patient's head to access the tumor. We then helped the surgeon attach the headpiece to a metal frame on the table so that it wouldn't move.

The surgeon then took electric clippers and carefully removed the hair around where he planned to make the incision. The remaining hair was parted away on all sides and he used tape to remove any loose pieces of cut hair from the area. We then prepped the scalp, being careful not to soak the surrounding hair with the alcohol solution and cause a potential fire hazard. The surgeon began the operation by cutting the scalp and carefully pulling back the flap of skin away from the skull. I know my mouth was open behind my mask; I couldn't look away! The surgeon then took a large drill bit and placed it on the skull to make the first entry into the hard surface. The loud buzzing lasted only a few seconds as fine pieces of bone dust whizzed from the tip of the drill. The drill bit had a special piece on it that let the surgeon know when the skull had been completely cut through so that he didn't keep drilling deeper and damage the brain. After taking this drill bit off, he took another special bit and made a larger cut in a semicircular shape. This bit also had a piece that kept the whirring drill bit from extending into the brain. In a few seconds, the surgeon had made a complete cut and carefully removed a piece of the skull about as big as the lid of a mason jar. The brain was right there now! The scrub tech placed the skull flap in a small bowl of saline on the back table.

The surgeon then carefully began moving away portions of the brain along certain anatomical separations. This was done slowly to prevent as much disruption as possible to the brain tissue. Eventually, the surgeon located the tumor and began the process of removing the tumor. After removing everything the surgeon thought was necessary, he began slowly removing all of the instruments and small cotton pads used to hold back the brain tissue.

The skull portion from earlier was taken out of the saline and the surgeon picked up a tray of small titanium plates and screws. He chose what he wanted and began screwing the plates onto the skull bone and reattaching it to the rest of the cranium. The skull piece was back where it started but now there was a thin outline of open space all around it. The skin flap was folded back and the surgeon began stitching the scalp. Soon the surgery was over. I was amazed.

My work was getting easier the longer I went in the rotations, I was doing well carrying over knowledge I was gaining with each service. However, I was still under preceptors and other nurses around me so I hadn't fully experienced a normal workload on my own yet. I left Neuro feeling more confident in my future in the OR. There was an opening on their team I was told as I finished my time with them and moved on to the final weeks of my training.

For my last rotation, I went to a much smaller rural hospital in the system that was about 45 minutes away from the main campus. There were only about 50 beds in the entire hospital if I remember correctly, so of course the OR was also very limited in size. There were four ORs, but the whole time I was there for my rotation, I only saw two or three rooms running at most. The schedule was almost always finished by 12 or 1 o'clock. They handled mostly general, ortho, and some eye cases. The surgical team members could handle whatever cases were on the board because they had to; no one worked in just one specialty. Many of the surgeries could be considered "outpatient" meaning most of the procedures were minor enough that the patients went home the same day or the very next day.

The atmosphere at this smaller hospital was very subdued compared to the bustling pace of the main campus hospital. The OR staff here did more background work than the nurses at the main campus. Some of them also ran the instruments themselves through sterile process-ing at the end of the day and they all pulled supplies and instruments for the next day's cases. The main hospital and many other ORs have staff to prepare case carts with instruments and supplies for the next day's surgeries so that the nurses and scrub techs can focus on patient care.

After this last rotation my training was basically over. It was time to find out the openings the system had and choose where I would begin working. Our group was gathered and we were all given a sheet with the openings. There were spots in General and Neuro at the main cam-pus, two spots at another hospital in the next suburb over that I hadn't been assigned to go to in my rotations, a few in the birth center(another place I hadn't gone; basically just doing c-sections), and surprisingly an opening at the rural hospital I just left. At this time the camaraderie our small group of new OR nurses had built was put on hold because now we all wondered if we wouldn't get the spot we preferred. Our training leader broke the ice as we si-lently viewed the openings and asked each of us what we we thought.

I certainly didn't want General, the birth center, or the rural OR. I hadn't even visited the other hospital where there were openings. I had really wanted Ortho! So far Neuro was my choice. I asked if I could take a day to go shadow at the other hospital. A few others also took the same opportunity to visit the places with openings that hadn't seen on their rotations. I went to the other hospital one day, which I saw was basically a smaller version of the main campus OR. They performed some ortho cases, but mainly general, urology, and some GYN. I didn't see anything that made me like or dislike anything compared to the places I had already been to, so it became my second choice behind Neuro.

I met with the Neuro coordinator as well as the main campus OR director for my interview. I wasn't nervous at all because I had already met these people and the questions were more specific about the time I had spent in Neuro and things related to their specialty. I also had done a brief interview during my shadow day at the other hospital but I really wanted Neuro at this point.

I had an idea of where my peers might want to go, but I wasn't the only one to have gone to Neuro. I was a little nervous because it wasn't a sure thing that I would get my first choice. That last week while we interviewed, we were placed in random specialties at the main hospital to simply observe and jump in to help where we knew we could. One by one, our leader came to each of us individually to offer us what was available. I was offered either an eight hour or ten hour shift in Neuro or an eight hour position at the suburb hospital. I chose the ten hour Neuro position, meaning I would work four ten hour shifts each week. I was so relieved to finally know where I would be starting. The other people landed in their first choices too, which I was glad for.

My training experience in hindsight went really well. We were given baby steps in the beginning while we adapted to the OR and its ways. We we placed with dedicated preceptors who we were with almost every day during our rotations. This was done so that the preceptor could keep a good measure of our progress and compare us to ourselves from one day to the next. If we had jumped from a different preceptor to the next every day, the preceptors wouldn't have really known how well we were advancing our knowledge. I also found out that the preceptors we had all had chosen to be preceptors, so they were invested in our learning and wanted to be active in teaching new nurses coming into the OR. There was a small pay bonus to being a preceptor, but I could tell that all the ones I had were knowledgeable and eager to pass on what they knew to us without the pay incentive.

We also got a wider perspective of the OR by going to multiple specialties for a few weeks at a time. This allowed us to see what the OR had to offer, but also the three week rotations let us stay in one place so that we could soak in the type of work each specialty performed. I couldn't imagine how confused a new OR nurse would be doing general cases one day, then ortho the next.

What I found was also unique to my training program was that at the end we were allowed to somewhat pick where we wanted to start. I think most ORs would want new people to work where their first choice is, but I've seen training programs at other hospitals place new people where the openings are regardless of if the person wanted to start there. It might be possible to switch specialties at a later time if openings occur, but this may take several months. Hopefully the nurse adapts and grows in their first specialty, but if not they may leave the OR altogether. I also understand the difficulty of an OR manager that has one Ortho opening and four new nurses want it. Three people will be getting their second or third choice. Our leaders were good about keeping our expectations realistic throughout the training regarding the openings available to us. They told us to keep an open mind and be willing to possibly start in a specialty that may not be your first choice.

The character traits that best suited me when I started in the OR through that training program were adaptability and perseverance. Walking into work having the mindset that the day you're about to have may be completely different than the one from yesterday helped me prepare for the unexpected. Yes, I may have been in a particular specialty, but sometimes cases get cancelled and an emergency surgery with other staff and surgeons flood into your assigned room and you must shift gears to accommodate the new situation. It's ideal for new OR nurses to have a consistent, repeatable workflow starting out so that they can build their foundation gradually. However this should also come with the expectation that the needs of patients and thereby the needs of the OR change and nurses must be ready to adapt to meet those changes.

Perseverance helped me in training as it did when I was first trying to break into the OR world. Every day in my training, and even for awhile when I was with my permanent specialty, I was meeting new people every single day. I didn't appreciate how exhausting this was, but I estimate I was meeting about 15 or 20 new people every week in the beginning. As odd as this may sound, it was a little tougher to remember people's names without glancing at their work badges because everyone in the OR is wearing the same scrubs, same hats, and same masks. This became easier the more I worked with the same people. I was also seeing procedures for the first time almost every day and the information was a lot to take in and retain. Sometimes I would encounter an impatient surgeon or nurse that had done a particular surgery "a thousand times" and they were irritated if I wasn't fast enough to get something. This happens to everyone just starting out and one mustn't let other people's impatience intimidate you in your learning. Eventually your perseverance pays off as you become a more seasoned OR nurse and things become easier, but you must endure the hard beginnings of all the new things you learn and experience.

Chapter 5. OR Culture

Many things in regards to the work environment of the OR are unique in my eyes compared to some of the other places I've worked. By now you've gathered what I have found to be rewarding about the job. Yet despite the interesting things I've seen and special people I've met, the OR is not all unicorns and rainbows. At the end of the day, it's still a job. It is common for me to look at my activity tracker after a 12 hour shift and see that I've walked 8 or more miles. If I'm on call, getting called back in to work with only two hours of sleep is really no fun. Even when I'm with a good-natured surgeon for the day and have enjoyable team members around, if the weather was nice I wouldn't turn down a chance to leave early for the day and steal an afternoon to play golf instead. I certainly carve out time for vacations and do my best to plan several consecutive days off to maximize my "work-life balance." If I get asked to work an extra shift I usually say no.

Anyone that gives an account of their workplace culture will probably share experiences revealing what they like and what they don't like. I will share some of my own and try to give a balanced perspective of what I've seen. Some of my experiences are humorous, some I look back on wistfully, and some I still get annoyed at today. I will share some stories that may seem random, but through them I hope you will get a better idea of the OR culture I've experienced.

I've already said that as much as is possible, surgeries are planned beforehand with good outcomes for the patients in mind. We prefer boring cases if it means the patient comes out on the other side better than when they came to us. If you want to come work in the OR thinking you will have heart-pounding excitement every day, you'd better look elsewhere. If emergencies roll into the OR people step up and deliver their best, but unless you work in a trauma center in a major city, this will probably not be your every day reality. When really sick patients are brought to us and we later find out they died in ICU the next day or only lived for a few more weeks, OR nurses feel sad because usually even in the brief time we saw them, we recognized that even the advancements in modern surgery wouldn't be enough for them to stave off the inevitable. At best, our actions may give them another few hours or days to say goodbye to their loved ones. Sometimes the extra three months a patient lives are worth the surgery they endure. I've experienced a few such times where we knew as we were setting up the OR room for surgery that death was coming for the patient soon, we were just delaying it as long as we could. The surgery was meant to alleviate as much pain in their final days as possible. In such times, a good surgeon would comment to the staff involved in the patient's care that their work was appreciated and helped the patient spend extra, precious time with their families. During such events, OR people grow closer together knowing they worked as a team to help another human's struggle against what eventually comes to us all.

I never expected working in the OR that I would end up listening to so many types of music I might have never otherwise heard or choose to listen to. Most surgeons want some type of music playing in the background during their operations and the styles of music you hear vary as much as the surgeons you work with. So far in my career, I've worked in four separate facilities with ORs and in every room there was either a sound system installed as part of the original design or a speaker system and player were set up on one side of the room. Some surgeons will bring their own wireless bluetooth speaker anyway along with their surgical loupes to their room and play music from their phones. The nurse is sometimes called upon to play DJ for the room if the surgeon gets bored with what's playing or if the surgeon has no particular preference, they just ask you to play something. In a challenging case they may ask for silence to concentrate better, but right after a timeout the surgeons want to hear their music as they are handed the scalpel. A chatty surgeon may pause their work and give unsolicited trivia about a particular song or band that is playing. Some surgeons like retelling interesting experiences they've had, so you might hear about them meeting someone backstage.

Generally speaking, if I am working with a new surgeon, I've been able to guess what they might prefer to hear based on the popular types of music that were around when they were in pre-med or med school. This isn't true for everyone, but it seems as I write this book in the year 2020, the doctors in their mid and late 40's gravitate toward 90's rock. The surgeons in their late 50's to mid 60's and older like the 80's and so on. However, the music choice I enjoyed best was from an older surgeon who played current alternative music from his XM Radio account. So you can't always use my age guide to anticipate what a surgeon may like. Just ask, or they'll let you know if you've chosen wrong!

I've heard country, heavy metal, hip-hop, classical, and

everything in between where the poppy "dentist office music" lives. It does get annoying hearing the same 90's pop song a few times a day. Not all surgeons mix up their playlists either and after a few weeks of working with them you find yourself memorizing the order of the songs playing. But at least if you're not enjoying the music one day, it's usually different the next. Overall the music has helped long days go by faster and I often jot down a song I've heard to add it to a playlist for myself later.

There was one surgeon I worked with often when I first started. For a few reasons, we just always tangled over something or another working together. I was either not fast enough for his taste in getting the OR ready for the next patient or he wouldn't do the necessary chart update or any number of other things that we sparred over. He was a country music aficionado that particularly liked George Strait. I don't love country music myself, but I'll admit George Strait is okay. One day, this doctor was really on my nerves. We didn't have a new instrument he had wanted because it hadn't been shipped to the hospital yet, so he had been snappy with me and other people all morning. As the first case started and the music played, he was chatting about every song or singing along. A popular George Strait song came on and the surgeon stepped back from the surgical field and sang a few lines. I really wished he would just shut up and work. I ran through some names of other musicians in my head before landing on a particular one. As he bent over to go back to work, I enthusiastically said, "Wow Doc, Willie Nelson is a national treasure!" I could see the fuses popping inside the doctor's brain as he looked up. His head turned sideways and he began blinking rapidly. He rested the instruments he was holding on the mayo stand. The metal pieces clanked as the unbelief at what I had just said washed over him. I had just quashed whatever remaining hope he had in his soul for my generation. "Willie Nelson? Are you shitting me?!?" He didn't even sound angry, just hurt. The older scrub tech standing across from him shot me a dirty look but simultaneously I could tell she was laughing on the inside. He sullenly went back to work and I could hear him swearing in a low voice to the scrub at the field. I also went back to my work without any more country music commentary the rest of the case to distract me from charting.

Where else but the OR can you see a 55 year old nurse with adult children scream out "DONE! DONE! ONTO THE NEXT ONE!!" along with the Foo Fighters after one case is over and she is cleaning an OR for another case? Another surgeon I remember had a way of asking for a particular device that is known as Gardner Wells traction tongs. When it was time for him to use it, he would croon, "let me see that tong...ba-beeee...that tong-a-tong-tong-tong!" to Sisqo's one hit wonder tune. Don't get me started on the number of times I've seen a co-worker twerk to whatever hip-hop beat is popular at the moment. We keep it professional when patients are around, but the sometimes intense nature of the OR is punctuated with light moments like these.

Can I tease the reps again? One year around Christmas time, my family had photos made for Christmas cards and we had some extra ones from our order. I had no plans to hand any out to my co-workers individually in the OR, but I did bring one to work a week after Thanksgiving and placed it by itself on a bulletin board in a common area. My friends complimented my family's picture when they saw me in the hall.

I was standing not far away from the board one day and two reps I hadn't met before saw the card and one asked the other, "who does he work for?" "I think he's the new Medtronic guy." I laughed as I walked by but didn't say anything as I continued my day. Maybe they didn't consider it was a nurse's family? Later that week, I saw two more Christmas cards next to mine and they were both from the families of the reps! When the following Monday came, by lunchtime there were five more Christmas cards around mine, all from various ridiculously good-looking reps and their families. None of my co-workers had brought any of theirs! Someone teased me why I wasn't wearing a red hat in the OR, I had apparently changed jobs and hadn't told anyone. Eventually some of my co-workers brought in cards of their own, but I guess the reps couldn't risk being left of of the Christmas card display.

Celebrating life events over food is nearly universal in the American workplace, and the OR is no different. The staff break room is often a place where you can find a cake someone has brought in for a birthday or a generous doctor has bought his room staff lunch that day. Whenever someone retires, there is usually a big send-off with a catered lunch or everyone brings something to share. At one place I used to work during the week of Christmas, the surgeons took turns ordering the whole staff delivery lunch each day. Pizza, Tex-Mex, Chinese, Greek, you name it. One year there was even catered ribs, macaroni and cheese, other side dishes, and pies. The poor patients who couldn't eat could all smell our food from down the hall. If you are trying to limit your intake, the OR can be a tough place to navigate.

In almost every OR I've seen, an hour or so is built into

the week's schedule to offer staff education or to make announcements with the whole OR present about new policies or things to be aware of. This usually happens for the first hour of the day on Wednesday mornings and the first cases start an hour later than usual. The reps sometime bring in breakfast for us on meeting days. As a rule, when they bring food it always has to accompany a staff training session about a new OR product or piece of equipment they are representing. There are many meeting days where I come in and there are huge bagels, donuts, or sausage biscuits. Coffee also, of course.

You are also sure to find at any given time a sign up sheet on a break room or locker room door for an outing at a local restaurant or some outing to recognize a peer's promotion or life event. Thursdays and Fridays are when people get their weekend plans together and before the last people are clocking out on Friday evenings, locations and times to meet at a downtown restaurant or bar are set. If you didn't make it or were on call that weekend, you get to hear the highlights on Monday morning.

Anyone who works in human resources or has managed people before know about the guideline to avoid conversations about religion and politics in the workplace. Contrary to this advice, both topics are often discussed, sometimes pointedly when five or more people are in the same room for several hours at a time. There's no way around it. When you work with people so closely and for so long, eventually some current event prompts a conversation about these things. I've seen grown adults maturely and tactfully discuss politics and religion without harming relationships. Such times can be stimulating and people can come away better informed.

I've also sadly seen others let differences affect them to the point of openly complaining to managers that they were stuck in OR rooms for the day with people they had become unfriendly toward due to differing political beliefs. This was acutely felt where I was working in 2016. Staff break rooms usually will have the news on the TV and sooner or later even it's local news, something polarizing comes on and people of all political stripes feel the need to offer their own commentary to whoever is present. Unfortunately, some people don't handle it well when they find not everyone agrees with their viewpoint.

Leading up to and after the 2016 election, the discomfort and angst among the staff was palpable for weeks where I was working at the time. I had my own opinions, but in the workplace where I spent so much of my time I couldn't allow those feelings to consume me. I had my job to do. I found myself leaving the room if a political discussion turned acrimonious, but being assigned to one OR for the whole day, that wasn't possible. It became maddening for me to listen to people argue constantly. No opinions were changed, only relationships divided. The hospital staff could be admonished by management to be professional, but only to a point. Some surgeons however, even if they were challenged to be more tactful in their conversations, had no filter and didn't care whether or not the staff they were with had differing opinions. It's one thing to disagree, it's another to mock and belittle work peers openly about who they voted for. People from both "sides" are guilty. I wish that those I worked with who were most vocal had not allowed current events to negatively affect work relationships with years of great teamwork behind them.

I'm pretty sure the big names in politics don't waste a minute wondering how workplace arguments about national politics play out. Of course they want your vote but they're not concerned about your relationships with co-workers over politics. If you work in the OR you will find very opinionated people, which is okay as long as things are kept professional. I know this atmosphere isn't unique to the OR, because I've heard similar things happen to friends in other completely different lines of work. I don't think future election years will be any different honestly, but at least management should try to foster a professional work environment if the conversations become personal and distracting from work.

On the other hand, discussions in the OR can also be extremely entertaining. I worked in a room one day where all the parties had a lively debate about whether or not we actually landed on the moon, along with other popular conspiracy theories. The scrub took the skeptic's approach while the surgeon was incredulous that anyone could doubt the success of America's space program. The scrub argued his points so thoroughly, and sometimes convincingly, that those who were present would sometimes be unable to challenge his arguments. We weren't sure if he was just playing devil's advocate or really believed what he was saying. We all left work that day in a lighter mood due the hilarious things he said about aliens and studio film sets of the moon.

We get to know the surgeons, and likewise they get to know the OR staff just as, if not better than their own families. We spend most of our time awake away from home in the workplace and the OR is no different. I've talked to the wives, husbands, or adult children of surgeons many times over the phone to relay personal messages if the surgeon was preoccupied. Over the years of meeting spouses at Christmas parties and talking about each other's families, the mutual familiarity grows. Many times while operating some surgeons will hash out disagreements they've had with their spouses or children to get advice on what to do next or seek validation from others for their perspective. After years of working with the same people, we become almost like each other's therapists or advisers. I've found that even though surgeons are in a class all their own due to the level of knowledge and training they've had, plus the much higher incomes compared to everyone else, we share many of the same life experiences. Their cars break down, they get the flu, they have personal relationship triumphs and setbacks. They feel satisfaction after a work day that goes smoothly and get frustrated when things go wrong.

On the outside looking in, yes surgeons can be intimidating due to the no-nonsense attitude they must have at times. Getting put on the spot by a surgeon can be very uncomfortable. As I gained more experience, I began to realize that almost every criticism I ever received from a surgeon was due to a shortcoming in my responsibility as a circulator or scrub, not an attack on me as a person. For example, if I didn't have a certain supply in the OR during a case that was necessary that I should have remembered and I needed to take 5 minutes to look for it, a surgeon might angrily chirp out, "come on, you know we need that!" They would say that to any circulator that forgot the item. You just remember next time and move on. Even still, you will run across some surgeons whose reputations notoriously precede them because they do have an air of superiority and they don't see the OR members as a team.

Such is life. I've found though that as long as I'm handling my responsibilities as a nurse, I can work around anyone else's bad attitude.

One certainly must have thick skin to work in the OR, and cannot be easily offended. There of course is conduct that is unacceptable and shouldn't be tolerated, even if "that's how they always are," is the excuse for someone behaving badly. I was told early on by a veteran OR nurse that you teach people how to treat you. If you permit yourself to be walked over by a pushy co-worker or rude surgeon, that's a sign to them it's okay to treat you that way from then on. It's intimidating for the first several months in the OR anyway, and in the beginning is when you start building your reputation. A new person needs strong self-esteem to begin with.

Even if someone's personality is "quiet", they need the self-confidence and ability to speak up when it is necessary. This can't be a trait that is gradually adopted, it must be there from the beginning. I've seen very smart, experienced nurses from other areas of the hospital leave the OR after only a few months because they couldn't handle being put on the spot in a room full of people when an important supply was missing or they accidentally contaminated something. Communication is often direct in the OR, and some people just do not adjust well to it.

To fully enjoy and contribute to the special culture of the OR, one must prove that they are competent. It's hard working with someone who constantly has to be reminded to do simple tasks or makes the schedule run behind because they forgot to do something. The first six months to a year is when a new nurse proves themselves in this way. Mistakes will happen, but the key is to let the consequence of a wrong action sink in and not allow it to repeat.

One time when I was in the training program, I wasn't paying attention to how close I was to a sterile table and my back side brushed up against the side of an instrument tray sitting on the edge. If you work in the OR long enough, you will accidentally contaminate something. The scrub barked at me to step away as she immediately picked up the tray and removed it from the field. I had to go find another tray and supplies and bring it back to the room as the scrub had to re-glove herself and set up an whole new back table. I actually wasn't sure if I had touched anything else since I had backed into the table, so a few hundred dollars worth of supplies had to be wasted and a new sterile table had to be opened. The monetary cost, the extra ten minutes to get more supplies, and the ire of the scrub were good motivations to make me pay much closer attention from them on to how close I was to a sterile field. I eventually regained the trust of the scrub I was with, but for the next few weeks she would stop working to watch me walk past her tables to make sure I didn't repeat my mistake.

In a perfect world, all the experienced people in an OR recognize when someone is new and will have patience with them as they grow. This isn't always the case and some impatient surgeons will be impatient no matter who the other people are in their room. Some experienced nurses that have seen almost everything and have a lot of advice to give instead choose to hold back their knowledge and let new people flounder and learn things the hard way unnecessarily. You may have heard the concept described as "eating their young." Some older nurses might say this is how they learned and treat new people coldly as an initiation. I've seen this changing in recent years for the better and it doesn't seem as prevalent. Of course, there will be ugly people regardless wherever one goes and the OR is no different. Be confident enough to speak up for yourself when you're not getting the answers you need and find the people who are willing to help; they are out there.

Not everything about OR culture appeals to everyone, but there is enough variety even within surgical workplaces for someone to find their own niche in which to flourish. An OR nurse can go to a large bustling trauma center with 30 or more ORs in a hospital that is world-renowned or find their place in a quiet outpatient surgery center with as few as two modest procedure rooms. Some people like their own specialty which they can work in every day for years and really master, or they can jump from Ortho to General to Neuro in the same week and become a jack of all trades. For anyone not wanting to stay locked into one workplace, travel nursing has become more prevalent in recent years. Hospitals will pay travel nurses handsomely to fill temporary or ongoing gaps in staffing to competent OR nurses. A nurse can spend a few months working in one place of the country while setting up their next destination several states away if they choose. Even within the specialty of OR nursing, there are many opportunities and settings where someone can find their home.

Chapter 6. Teaching And Precepting

I mentioned earlier that I had interviewed for an OR that didn't accept me, and years later ended up sitting on the other side of the interview table of the very same hospital. This change occurred when I became a clinical educator in the OR and one of the tasks was interviewing people that would be accepted to that hospital's OR training program. It was a very satisfying feeling when the disappointment I felt that day years ago after being rejected became a sense of accomplishment as I interviewed people whose place I had been in years before. That letdown years ago had been temporary and after proving myself in the OR, I had been chosen to help pick who I thought could handle the job. By the time I made it to this role, thankfully there were new people there alongside me who conducted interviews more professionally.

I was sought out for the teaching job due to something I thought was insignificant but turned out to be the main reason I was asked to interview. About two years into my first OR job, I was asked to join the education committee for the entire OR. There were about eight nurses and scrub techs on this committee and they met each month to discuss and plan the weekly education staff meetings for the OR. Someone from my specialty had retired and her spot on the committee was vacant. I reluctantly agreed because honestly I didn't necessarily want to do more work without more pay. I realized after a few meetings that I was wrong to feel this way because I had input into what the staff needed for education and I had the chance to occasionally speak in front of the whole OR staff during staff meetings and get better at public speaking. My major contribution from my time on this committee was creating a one hour presentation with one of our main surgeons for him to present to the main OR one morning. Because I was familiar with his work and also what the main OR would expect to hear about neurosurgery from a nursing standpoint, I was able to determine how best to guide his talking points. Everyone who attended received a continuing education credit and I think everyone benefitted from the experience. I added this part of my work experience to my resume and someone at the other hospital came across it for something unrelated and decided to reach out to me about an open position with the education team. I interviewed for the spot and was offered the job! Something I thought was minor led to a very unique role I had not expected. I also received a significant pay increase when I switched to this role. The moral of the story is don't refuse to contribute to your workplace in extra ways because you never know where it might lead!

I'll write what I've learned about teaching others, but I certainly don't have all the answers to the many challenges that education brings. I say this because I have spent less time as an educator as I have as an OR nurse, and I've moved onto other roles since then. I am still learning what works and what doesn't when it comes to effectively teaching people with different backgrounds and learning styles. However, I can certainly share what my experiences have been thus far. Maybe new people just starting in the OR and even those in management can learn something from successes and mistakes I've made.

Interviewing candidates is how you find new people

to train in the first place, so I'll start there. People that interview potential candidates for a training program are looking for qualities they know they will need to succeed in the OR. Among other things, the major qualities we always looked for was someone's sense of self confidence, willingness to learn, and whether or not they would work well within a team. All of the standard professionalism traits were still assessed but those were three that stood out to us. It was also easier to tell who was really interested in the OR based on how much they knew about it from prior experiences or seeking out knowledge about the OR. For example, if we asked someone why they were interested in the OR, if they said something along the lines of "oh, I really like Grey's Anatomy and I think I want to try OR nursing," we saw this as a red flag. Whereas if someone had shadowed in the OR before or was impressed after some nursing school clinicals, we at least knew they had been in an OR before and had a idea of what it was like. Some people also showed the level of their interest based on whether or not they had sought out more information on their own about the OR. Maybe they read some books about the OR(like this one!) and wanted to take the steps to begin a new career in the OR.

Choosing who interviews potential new people can also be important to picking staff who will be a good fit for the OR. Some ORs only have the director or a coordinator conduct interviews. I think ideally a director/manager, coordinator, educator, and a trusted frontline OR nurse should conduct interviews to get a good first impression of a potential OR nurse. Any more than two or three people conducting an interview can become nerve-wracking for the candidate, so a combination of a director/manager, educator, coordinator, or staff nurse could be considered.

Those in management and staff education have certain qualities they look for in someone, but I think you also need the perspective of a nurse who is in the room every day with surgeons and patients. Giving a nurse a say in who works alongside them can be rewarding, but that person also needs to be responsible enough to shoot straight with a new person while also recognizing potential in them. People in managerial roles have important responsibilities, and they usually have had years of frontline experience behind them, but they can forget what the daily grind is like and they need to hear a voice from someone in that role. When I first became an educator, I stopped direct patient care and in a few months I had adjusted to my new workflow that didn't include the every day tasks I used to do as an OR nurse.

I wish I had some secrets to share about how to make sure someone picks only those people who will stay in the OR for years and years and become great OR nurses. Unfortunately, I saw some people who had great interviews drop out of the OR after only a year while some don't even make it out of the training program. Some people that leave say they missed more face-to-face patient care and didn't appreciate how little they do talk to the patient. Some people who are very intelligent and pick up new ideas and concepts quickly get spoken to harshly a single time by a surgeon or co-worker and they never regain their confidence. They decide to go back to what they did before because even if a bad situation is addressed and resolved, they don't want to feel under that type of pressure in the workplace. I've seen a few good nurses find out at the end of the training program that they wouldn't be able to start in their favorite specialty and proceed to meltdown about their futures in the OR. They weren't able to see beyond the next six months or a year and realize they don't have to stay in one specialty forever. On the other hand, there are those we may have been unsure about through the training and they turn out to be some of the best nurses in the OR.

By this point, I've detailed how the OR can be very challenging for new people to adapt to. Not only are the nursing responsibilities different than what someone might expect, a new person still has all of the normal things to adjust to in a new workplace. Clocking in, meeting new people, and just getting acclimated in general are things to adjust to on top of the new things they are learning about the OR. Even an experienced OR nurse needs time to learn the workflow and learn where important supplies, instruments, and equipment are. For the first several weeks, a new person in the OR needs a lot of support and should be slowly introduced to new challenges. Whoever is in charge of scheduling staff for OR assignments every day shouldn't put someone into a difficult surgeon's room the first day for example. Ideally the first few days and weeks are spent working similar cases so that the new person can see the same tasks over and over and develop confidence with each passing success before moving on to more challenges. The healthcare adage of "see it, do it, teach it" applies in the OR, but the middle action should be repeated several times before moving on to more challenging tasks. Familiarity with regular tasks needs to be ingrained before adding new things to learn. This builds confidence and lets the new person get a strong footing before moving on to something else.

Along with training new people goes choosing the right preceptors to bring them into the fold. It's best to choose preceptors with experience, which in my opinion should be one full year at minimum. If that even sounds too low, I agree. In a perfect world, it's at least two or three. However that may be the only option in some settings. A solid OR nurse, even at one year, might have a better perspective to share with a new person because it wasn't so long ago for them that they were learning how to adjust to the OR. They will remember what it was like to start out better than someone who has been there for ten or more years and may have more understanding of what the new person is going through. Older nurses will certainly have more experience to pass along, but may be more prone to impatience with new people because they are so far removed from their first days.

For myself and many people I've talked to, a new OR nurse doesn't feel truly independent until 6 months to a year on their own. For me this meant I'm not calling my coordinator/charge nurse every few hours asking for help finding a supply or how to order a blood delivery from the blood bank. To try putting a new OR nurse with someone who only has six months of experience themselves doesn't do either person credit. You may think this seems obvious, but I've seen managers do it it all the time! Let the new nurses under a year learn on their own and don't put people in their rooms to shadow or precept. A nursing student or potential hire need to be placed with experienced people that won't be distracted or flustered by someone watching them or asking questions about their job.

It may go without saying, but preceptors need to *want* to be preceptors. An experienced nurse may have all the knowledge necessary to pass onto someone new, but if they don't have a personality that is conducive to a good teaching relationship, they will not help new people adapt the way they should. There should be a universal expectation in any OR that if a new person, or even someone experienced just asking for help will get assistance from the experienced people when they need it. A preceptor-trainee relationship however requires an ongoing, dedicated interaction that allows honest discussion and feedback. Every time a new person has a problem, they need to know their preceptor is always available to help. To have this, the preceptor needs to be approachable and patient so that the new person will be comfortable in learning from them.

Ideally, a trainee stays with their preceptor for at least two or three weeks before moving on to another specialty or preceptor. Having the same person assessing them means the trainee can be looked at over a period of consecutive work shifts. Good habits and bad habits can be picked up on and addressed more immediately than if someone is constantly passed back and forth among multiple preceptors. Anyone can have a bad day in the OR whether it's forgetting some supply, insufficient charting, or being unable to anticipate the next task. If someone keeps having the same issues, the preceptor will be able to catch those things within the same week. If a trainee has a different preceptor everyday and is struggling with something, that problem may fly under the radar for weeks and that bad habit becomes harder to break. I've seen both methods used, and I think having the same preceptor for two weeks or more make much more sense than randomly picking a different preceptor off the board every day for a new person.

When a new person is brought into the OR, it's important for the preceptor to introduce their trainee to as many people as they can. With everyone wearing the same scrubs and wearing hats and masks, it's not as easy to learn who is who in the beginning as it might be in other settings. A new person as well as the preceptor need to be upfront with the people they work with about the trainee's level of experience so that realistic expectations are set. A surgeon and scrub team *should* be more patient with someone who is seeing a particular surgery for the first time versus someone who might be new to the workplace but has ten years of OR experience and thus should already have an expectation of what the OR is like. An introduction with a new person could go something like this: "Dr. Smith, this is Karen, she's a nurse from the training program, she's been in the OR for two weeks, so we're still learning how to circulate." It should also be impressed upon trainees to speak up for themselves whenever they are in a situation they haven't seen yet or meeting someone new. Even experienced nurses with several years behind them might be asked at times to assist in other types of surgeries they may not be as familiar with, and they need to speak up and ask for assistance from others in the room who do have that knowledge. New nurses need to learn how to advocate for themselves from the beginning because it's something they will always need to do.

At the end of each week or even each shift, the preceptor and trainee should set aside at least five minutes or more to talk about what is going well and what needs improvement. It's best to also have a written progress report where both people can place their input and discuss what is happening. Whether this is done after every shift or just every week is up to the people responsible for training new staff. The important thing is that whatever events are happening are documented and discussed so that there is a record of how well or how poorly the trainee is progressing. Their training can be seen from its beginning through until the end. Whoever oversees the training of new people can look at the data to see what training practices are benefiting new people the best and what might need attention.

When I first became a clinical educator, I underestimated how daunting it could be to stand in front of a group of a dozen or more people and give a one hour lecture on an OR-related topic. I had always felt comfortable when I was a front line nurse explaining something to one or two other people as long as I understood it myself. The public speaking aspect of the role was something that I had to adjust to. The actual nervousness wasn't the biggest issue, it was the feeling that I didn't want people leaving the lecture confused or lacking in what they needed to know when it was over. I worried most about them not retaining important information they would need later. I also didn't want to just read Power Point slides and drone on about the basic information; I wanted them engaged and able to relate to what I was teaching. Having spent the first two thirds of my life in a classroom of some kind, I knew what good teaching and bad teaching looked and sounded like.

I was given a few months to prepare my first lectures to the upcoming OR training class. I inherited a few topics from the person whose spot I replaced on the team of educators. Some co-workers suggested that rather than rely on the notes the last person had made with their presentations, I study the topics and create my own slides in their own order. This would help me so that as I went through them, I could more easily speak about each one because

I would be the one who had arranged them in the first place. I also studied the specific hospital policies related to each topic and placed the key points along the way in the lecture. Another co-worker gave me the pointer to try to relay an event from my own work history that applied to the material whenever I could so that the listeners could get examples of real-world situations. I also found later this would make me more relatable as a presenter and help create a more open dialogue with students later on in other teaching settings.

I went to work arranging my presentations and mapping out the order in which I wanted to present the material. The general rule I followed for each slide was to give myself 30 seconds to a minute and a half per slide to talk about it before moving on to the next one. There's no professional standard to this concept that I'm aware of; I just wanted to have a consistent length of time per slide so that I didn't initiate "death by power point" by throwing 80 slides at a class for a 45 minute lecture, nor did I want to cram several paragraphs into single slides and make the material overwhelming. I tried to keep keywords and phrases clear and simple on the screen while verbally ad-libbing the thoughts behind each one.

For each presentation, I had a printed out version in front of me with a single slide on it and some handwritten key trigger words or short hints for myself that weren't on the actual slides. I did this so that if I needed I could be reminded of something to talk about pertaining to the current slide without merely reading word for word off the screen on the wall, which anyone can do. I always felt this was a minor distraction because I would always have to flip the page in my stack as I clicked the mouse or pointer remote to move to the next slide, but for me just starting out, it was all I needed to quickly arrange my thoughts. The few seconds of pause was all I needed to collect myself and begin a new train of thought. I always admired peers of mine who had already been teaching for years that could stand next to the screen itself and not rely on notes to prompt them to say what came next.

I would add pictures to the presentation whenever I could to further illustrate certain things and also brought in physical items to pass around whenever I could. For example, it's much easier to show someone the differences in all the types of suture there are when they can see for themselves with their own eyes. I would scout the OR every few months for expired suture packages that had been set aside and save them for upcoming classes. The visual and tactile methods were almost always well-received because merely listening and reading material can only go so far. Plus, passing around items helped fill the time allotted as I continued talking about the material at hand.

In the few weeks leading up to my first time teaching, I found an empty conference room in the hospital and literally practiced nearly word for word what I wanted to say just to see if I was going to adequately fill the time. I stood at the front of the room and went through each slide, talking to myself as the timer on my phone ran. Hearing my words out loud helped me discover a few things to adjust in the presentations after I was done and I could hear my own speaking tempo moving through the material. If I was short five or ten minutes, I would add back in two or three slides of content I might have cut that I thought would be helpful. If I was over, I usually left the presentation alone because I still had a tendency to talk fast, and I knew I could still cover the material if need be. I left five minutes per hour at the end of my allotted time for questions.

I won't lie, I was very nervous the first few times I taught. I just wanted to do a good job and make the time I had worthwhile to the students. Luckily, the teaching evaluations that the class would fill out after each lecture were mostly positive and encouraging. Even after teaching the same lectures a few times, I would notice a few minor things that I would need to adjust. After teaching the first six times or so, I began to settle in to the role of talking out loud for long periods of time. I found that I always liked having water nearby, even if I didn't need it. Sometimes I would take a sip just to give the class and myself a break from the cadence of my voice and take a chance to reset my next thought internally before speaking again.

In the half hour right before I would teach even after I had been doing it for months, I would be very anxious and I could feel my heart racing. I just wanted to walk right into the room and get started to quell the nerves. The educator before me probably wouldn't have appreciated that, so I would simply review the first five slides slowly to myself and practiced slow breathing exercises to calm down before I went into the classroom. Usually, the class was given a short five or ten minute break between each lecture, so I would also get that short time to myself to bring up the presentation on the screen and collect myself at the teaching podium as the class sipped their coffees and meandered in and out of the classroom during the break. When everyone was back, I would take a deep breath and go. In a class of 12-15 people, there were a few that locked eyes with me through the entire lecture, a few that mostly looked at the screen or at their notes, and a few who had their phones out basically the whole time. It felt odd calling out people who were my age and even older to pay attention, but we would have to do it from time to time. We always tried not to embarrass anyone, but what we were teaching was important and anyway it was rude of them to ignore the time we had to teach them.

For certain topics, our teaching supervisor would arrange for other people to come present what they were best suited to teach. We would have an organ donor representative from our state organization come for an hour and talk about organ donation and what the process looks like for staff in the OR. In our particular hospital, we might go months without an organ donor case and not everyone does them enough to know what people should be taught about the process. The person that works with it every day was best suited to present that knowledge, not an OR nurse who might have only done one or two donor cases in their past. Certain product representatives also might come to give more in-depth discussions about particular surgical products that the nurse would later see in use. A practice we also began to adopt in the latter part of my teaching days was bringing in coordinators or charge nurses from certain specialties in the OR to present overviews of common procedures that were unique to their specialty. We had the General team coordinator discuss laparoscopic cholecystectomies and colon resections. The Neuro coordinator discussed craniotomies and spinal fusions. Each coordinator would discuss the main surgeries their team worked on every week and brought instruments and equipment with them to present. This was a good way for the new students to get a deeper look into each of the specialties and also get to know the coordinators to whom they might later report to in their work roles.

We also had members from each role in the OR come to the class and give a brief ten or fifteen minute talk about their job. Radiology technicians, nurse anesthetists, surgeons, scrub techs, cleaning staff, secretaries, basically anyone we thought the new nurses should hear from came to talk about themselves and their place in the OR. This was also a great way to foster teamwork and get the new people acclimated to where they fit in the OR and what others around them in the workplace brought to the table. Many of these people shared their educational backgrounds and what they liked most about the OR. The students could ask questions in a setting that was "off the record" and the people we chose were certainly willing to talk candidly about things that might bug them in their work load and how nurses could help or hinder their jobs. The surgeons were always sure to mention that they liked quick turnovers between cases. The cleaning staff always appreciated extra help cleaning the rooms if nurses could return after taking their patients to PACU. The common theme we always came across in these talks was communication and how it could make or break an OR.

We were fortunate enough as educators to have lots of equipment and supplies at our disposal to help teach the nurses how to properly do things such as sterile gowning and gloving, setting up a back table full of instruments, draping, prepping, passing instruments back and forth, and many other things that are best done by actual practice. Lectures and even passing items around the room only went so far; on the days we spent time practicing actual skills you could see the so-called light bulbs coming on with each student all day long. The classes's confidence grew as they were able to practice these skills without the nervousness of other people watching them in a real setting. Of course the first time they did these tasks in real situations with other nurses and doctors watching them they were anxious, but by then they had performed the skills several times already in practice and it wasn't so nerve-wracking.

We structured our training program into two main parts. The class would spend the first four weeks mainly in the classroom and skills lab, and two months of clinical with dedicated preceptors in the actual OR. In the classroom portion, the class had three or four days of lecture and one full day of observation-only "clinical" in the OR on the Friday of each week. The first two weeks of this classroom portion were heavy on lecture while the last two weeks were spent more on practicing skills and listening to people besides the educators teach them about the OR. This was when the product representatives and other members of the OR team would come talk to the class. On each observation day, a student was placed with a trusted OR nurse and they were told to focus on seeing the things they had learned about in lecture that week. They were encouraged to ask questions and if the OR nurse guiding them felt it was appropriate, they would allow the student to perform tasks in the room. We liked to see people take initiative and try to help the staff in their room to the best of their ability, but we didn't have an expectation for them to take over the job of the circulator based on only a few days of lecture. The time for added responsibility would come later in the clinicals.

We tested the knowledge of the students using computerized testing on the lecture material. Out of fifteen or so lectures, five or six questions were picked from each one to place on the test. A surgical instrument test was also given where the students walked into a classroom with surgical instruments laid out on the table with numbers next to them and they had to fill in the blank of what the instrument was. The passing grade for these tests was 80%. We also had skills check-offs like in nursing school to assess if the student could perform basic OR skills correctly. These skills covered scrubbing, gowning and gloving, setting up a sterile table, draping, passing instruments, and so on. After passing these tests, part two of the training program began with clinicals.

The clinical portion of the training program was spent almost completely in the OR itself. Each student spent two weeks at a time with the same preceptor in the same service before moving on to a different specialty. The student could get a better feel for the type of cases in each specialty as well as get to know the staff and surgeons a little more consistently. Our team of educators were assigned two or three students and everyday we would check in on them for at least ten minutes just to maintain contact and be a resource for them. On the Friday afternoon of every week, the students gathered for an hour and everyone was given the opportunity to talk about the things they had seen. These debriefing sessions were good for people to talk about their experiences so that they could all see that they were not alone in feeling overwhelmed. They could also share things they were getting better at. The educators would also talk to the preceptors to see how well their trainees were adapting and progressing. Usually if someone was having an issue, we could learn about it fairly soon and address it. The first few weeks were stressful to the students because they were first putting into practice the things they had learned. For the most part though, each week brought added confidence and the educators felt less and less inclined to check up on them the longer clinicals went on.

Occasionally, a few students would not improve upon their experiences as time went on and many times they left the program completely. They usually went back to their prior nursing job or found another floor in the hospital. As a group, my team felt regret if someone didn't complete the program because it meant one less person would be in the OR. We would wonder aloud what we could have done differently with those specific people to help them stay. Ultimately though we understood that the OR simply isn't for everyone and it's best to find that out early on rather than stubbornly trying to make it work.

On the last week of the clinicals, the openings on each specialty were revealed to the class and interviews began. We had the OR director, team coordinator, and an educator talk with each person about their interests. At this point, it wasn't really an "interview," by now everyone was familiar with each other. It was more of a conversation about where the student felt they would fit the best just starting out. Unfortunately, there weren't always enough openings if several people wanted the same specialty. Some people understood this and went with their second choice. I wish I could say all of these people who had to accept their second choice adapted well to their teams, but even after a few months sometimes they would transfer to other surgical teams and find better fits or leave the OR altogether.

The things that were most appreciated from the people we taught was being willing to listen and being available to talk to about their concerns. Being able to do this meant us as educators being visible and present in the OR. We all had an office where we worked, but we almost always dressed in OR scrubs in the event we need to go to the OR for something. Looking at the daily schedule and walking down the halls helped us stay present in the OR environment, even if we weren't directly responsible for patients. Even helping position a patient for surgery only took a few minutes and made it easier for us to talk to staff. Having already been an OR nurse for years let me know in what ways I could help the nursing staff without getting in the way of their workflow. Many educators I know also work an occasional part time shift to keep up their clinical experience and also have more income. I encourage any clinical educator to do their best to keep their finger on the pulse of the workplace they support. All nurses have a responsibility to educate and help new people in the OR, I was fortunate to spend some of my career doing it full time.

PART TWO

Stories

Chapter 1. The Smell of a Nurse in the Morning

I stood still on the shiny waxed floor, looking up at the three large screens angled down from the wall next to the coordinator's desk behind me. One of the TVs would have been very suitable for our break room, but then again the only thing people seem to want to watch in the hospital are the mundane morning talk shows and local news. Besides, these screens are "medical-grade," which we were told can handle the rigorous environment of the hospital and therefore cost almost twice as much as the regular ones from the box store down the street. Yes, the screens hanging on the wall indeed could handle the fine accumulating dust on their top surfaces throughout the year. They were, after all, cleaned about twice a year whenever the surveyor teams would arrive with clipboards. Instead of showing me hungover musicians from a band lip-syncing their hit single to a 7 am street audience in New York City, or the local weatherman telling me about the 30% chance of rain this afternoon, I saw the names of surgeons and procedures and times in lines down the "board." Although the screens possessed the latest visual technology, they were still called the board in the operating room because that's what they used to be: chalkboards in the early days, then dry-erase boards with markers and magnets. The name remained even when hospitals began using the screens. Everyone in the operating room no matter their role, education, or experience stopped by the board throughout the day to see where and when they were expected to go.

One of my fists rested against my hip, the other held a small white foam cup half-filled with pebbled ice and tap water that was getting colder with each sip as the water to ice ratio began to favor the ice. I sniffed the familiar foam smell that thousands of others in the hospital and in workplaces everywhere recognize. "Do they actually think getting rid of our cups will save the hospital that much money?" I thought as I scanned the board, giving each line no more than a few seconds to stick in my memory before moving to the next. A rumor had been started earlier in the week that the hospital was going to stop providing the bulk packaged 8 ounce foam cups to our break room. Most people seemed to have their own mug or trendy metal tumbler stashed away in the break room somewhere it seemed. Maybe the hospital wanted something else "medical grade" and axing our mass-produced foam cups was the next target. It could even be part of a "green" initiative to tell the media about! I would cave and get a tumbler if it came to that. This morning, I had my 8 ounces of water like always and no more, because an 8:30 break might really be a 10:30 break and a circulator isn't allowed to leave their team for something unrelated to the case, even something as personal as a pee break.

My weight shifted to the left, then balanced in the middle, and to the right as I looked at all of the words. My shoes didn't squeak on the floor like some of my co-workers around me as they shuffled into the space where the board was. I had fresh shoe covers on, I could walk the long hallways of the OR quietly while others could be heard before they could be seen, sounding like they were walking across a basketball court, but without the sharp rubber chirps that players make during a game. I preferred my quiet but fast gait, the shoe covers' thick papery surface kept me from squeaking but they also kept blood and bits of tissue from between the crevices in my sneakers, at least until the end of the day when they had worn through and I needed a fresh set. Some people simultaneously pulled their surgical hats and masks from bins nearby as they searched for their names and where they were going to spend the next 8-12 hours. Others that were still in commuting mode rushed past the board without a glance and went straight to the locker room to change. They had clocked in just in time. Soon we would all be wearing the same clothes, even if some were wearing the wrong sizes. The same people began arriving at the board that always arrived at this time of the morning. The night shift nurse coordinator sat back in the office chair watching us walk up. She was giving the day shift coordinator a recap of the night's events. An anesthesiologist and a surgeon were discussing a patient's background and whether or not surgery remained in their near future this morning. The small area began to fill with people.

I sensed someone standing right behind me. They were very close. A raspy but quiet noise of someone breathing deeply was behind my right shoulder. The odor of her morning cigarette filled the air around me. Another stepped closely to my left and the side of her arm touched mine. After the contact, she didn't move away. I instinctively inched forward away from the breathing and the touching. Old Smokey 's mouth whispered in my ear, "don't move, we're smelling you."

The pervy old women shared a burst of laughter between themselves as the winced look on my face revealed my disgust. I shook my head and turned around to face them both, my initial shock wearing off as I tried to form the words of a comeback. "Who says that?!," I thought. I began to laugh myself at the audacity of the salty OR veterans. "I'm glad I could be here for you this morning," was all I could manage in response. A whiff of my morning shower's body wash was all it took to get teased by some women old enough to be my mother. The nurse at the desk laughed at my blushing as I made my way around the others looking at the board. "Looks like you're starting to fit in," she said as she handed me a printed schedule for the day. I had been an OR nurse for about six months.

Chapter 2. Lace By The Fireplace

Dr. Williams was one of the older surgeons out of the group that I worked with most often. He was polite to his patients, polite to staff(when the schedule was running on time), and very polite to a few select CRNAs who always seemed to be assigned to his cases. He was divorced, and although I hadn't known him back when he was married, older nurses told me he had been a terror to work with, especially when the divorce was happening. They said that nowadays his mood was the best it had ever been.

He had a surgeon's demeanor that was not unusual: reasonable and steady when things were going according to plan, but he could have a short fuse whenever he had to repeat himself or was made to wait longer than what he thought was appropriate. He might start out the day with you cordially, but if something was missing from his OR that was needed, he could blow his stack instantly. The very next minute, he would be telling you a joke he had heard over the weekend or ask you how your kids were doing. When I first began working with him, this dynamic was jarring because I never felt at ease. Eventually, I learned how to maneuver a work day with Dr. Williams without upsetting his particular expectations.

One of the quirks about Dr. Williams was that he wanted to know every single thing that came across his phone during a surgery. Obviously a patient update from the floor or a message from his office were important things to pass along, but he even wanted to read every single text, stock market update, and weather alert that popped up. This could be so annoying because I would have to stop my charting or stop another task during the case to access his phone and either walk it over to him to look at or announce what it was that came across his screen. If it was just a news update or something trivial, he might just say "ok thanks" and not miss a beat working. A text though either had to be read aloud or walked over to him to see. Every notification made a single ping and the volume had to be turned up so it could be heard, nothing could be left to check on after the case. After the first week working with Dr. Williams, I had memorized the access code to his phone like all the other nurses. I knew it by heart just like I knew the number to our OR front desk and PACU.

One day, I had finished a few morning cases with another surgeon and their room was done for the day by early afternoon. Dr. Williams was in another room and the nurse who had been with him was leaving for the day and I was sent in as her replacement. I entered the room and immediately saw one of the CRNAs who worked with Dr. Williams seemingly all the time. She was attractive, 45, fit, and also divorced. Her bottom scrubs were super tight and her top was one size larger due to her enhanced… physique. Her eyes peeked over the drape at Dr. Williams and they were talking about a particular resort in the Caribbean they had both been to. The air was heavy with flirtatious banter. "Haha, oh Dr. Williams, you'll have to tell me the next time you go, I can show you that island with the hidden lagoon." The scrub glared at him out of his view as he stood back from the field to chat with the CRNA. It was clear they had been talking all day. I gestured like I was about to vomit and the scrub gave a quick nod and made her eyes open big to affirm my assessment of the room.

As it turned out, this was one of my call days. I had to work my normal 12 hour shift but also be available to work until 7am the following morning if an emergency came up. As it also turned out, Dr. Williams was the on-call surgeon that evening. We finished the case I had given relief on by late afternoon and the schedule was empty, no more cases! I went to the break room for a few minutes but soon the OR charge nurse called me to say Dr. Williams had an add-on case. I groaned and the scrub who was with me exclaimed, "great, more smoochy-smoochy time with 'Boobalicious' and Dr. Williams." I was just irritated I would have to stay late; the case was going to take at least three hours to prepare for and complete. I wasn't going to leave until probably 9 I thought. We picked ourselves up and got the room ready to go.

I found out it wasn't even an urgent case, just one that Dr. Williams hadn't wanted to wait to do the next day. I was even more pissed! The CRNA came bouncing into the OR; wouldn't you know she was on call too. "I'll be in holding when you're ready," she said as she grabbed her meds from the anesthesia cart and left the room. "She'll be in holding when you're ready," the scrub said in a sugary voice as the door closed. I rolled my eyes and kept working. "At least there's the overtime," I reminded myself.

The case started and we began working like it was any other case. The flirty comments continued back and forth between surgeon and CRNA. The case was going smoothly, and it looked like we might finish a little sooner. Dr. Williams was becoming more edgy though as the evening progressed whenever his phone pinged. Doctors don't like being on call any more than nurses do. Whatever good-natured talk he was having with the female at the head of the room shifted to barely-controlled annoyance whenever the phone interrupted. Sure enough, a text came through from the ED that I immediately recognized would be our next add-on case. I showed it to Dr. Williams. "DAMMIT!!!" We all sighed. He turned away and went back to operating. A few minutes later: ping! He angrily slammed a needle driver onto the mayo stand. "WHAT NOW?!?" It was a text from "Mindy." "When will you be off?" I read to him from the phone. Dr. Williams growled, "I'll handle that later" and went back to finishing the surgery.

Luckily, the add-on case probably wasn't going to take very long, but by the time we finished that case, turned over the room, and the next patient was draped and prepped, it was close to 10 pm. I was so tired. Everyone else was too. We had all been working since 7 that morning. We dutifully carried on with the work. The doctor had become growingly impatient ever since we knew about the extra case. In the day time when an add-on case happens, someone is almost always available to pick supplies and instruments so that when the OR is cleaned, the staff can immediately begin opening the materials needed for the case. The scrub and I had to do this ourselves however, which took an extra ten minutes. Dr. Williams even came to the room between the cases and tried hurrying us along, but he grudgingly recognized that we were short-handed and he sullenly went back to the doctor's lounge to await his time.

Just a few minutes after we began this case we all hoped was the last one for the night, the unmistakable, dreaded ping from the phone struck the room again. Dr. Williams just kept his head down and silently shook it side to side, grimly waiting to see what was in store. The scrub sighed. The bubbly CRNA was tapped out. The flirting was over, she had exhausted all of her charms at this point.

The name "Mindy" was on the home screen. I punched in the pass code as I had done so many times that day. The phone immediately opened Mindy's thread, and in my head I said who the text was from, but in reality I didn't, and couldn't speak. It was a photo of a woman's butt draped in green turquoise lingerie. The dimly lit room with a fireplace in the background revealed the nearly naked backside of Mindy, who was also wearing knee high black leather boots. Mindy's hands were clutching the mantle above the fireplace in front of her and half of her face leered at me from behind her long, dark blonde hair falling over her back and shoulders. The upper piece of the lingerie tightly contained the rest of Mindy, except for the muffin top that she wasn't able to fully conceal with the contorted pose she made. She had typed "waiting for you..." below the cursed image.

I tried to recognize who it was. I didn't know a Mindy in the OR. Was Mindy at Dr. William's house? Her place? Was she his girlfriend? Ex-wife? A hooker? These questions struck me all at once as the image burned itself into my tired mind. "What is it?!" I think I heard. I could feel my mouth open and stretch against the mask tied to my face. I wasn't making a sound. I stood there holding the phone and looked up at Dr. Williams. I couldn't walk it over to him, the scrub might see it. "Uhh.." I managed to say. The surgeon spun around and glared at me. I motioned for him to walk over. "SERIOUSLY?!? JUST TELL-" he yelled as he took the three steps to stand where I was holding his phone. The rest of his words froze as he saw what I had seen. "From Mindy," I said smugly. Our eyes met. Two men looked at each other and in those few seconds a clear understanding passed between us without a word being said. We could only see half of each other's faces, Mindy too looked up at us from my hands in her partially hidden gaze.

"I see." A brief pause followed. "I'll see about that later." I pressed the phone on its side and the screen went black. The doctor turned around quietly and walked back to his place by the patient. The scrub peered at me sideways. "Not an add-on," Dr. Williams flatly said, knowing she was trying to determine what I had seen. I shook my head and raised my hand in a stopping motion to signal now wasn't the time. Not another word came from the doctor and not another sound came from the phone for the next thirty minutes. The surgery ended.

The scrub and I met each other almost at the same time at the scrub machine to ditch our work outfits and finally head home. We saw Dr. Williams walking fast down the hallway away from the OR. He hadn't even changed out of his scrubs. "Stay warm tonight Doc" I said. He shot me a glance but kept trucking. I caught a sly grin on his face at the last second as he departed from earshot. "What was that all about?" I told the scrub all about it as we walked out of the unit and we laughed all the way to the parking deck. It was almost midnight.

Chapter 3. Birthday Cake

I slammed the foley kit into the round trash can next to me. The dark yellow-brown betadine from the kit splashed up and over the edge of the can and landed in spots on the floor. "FINE!" I yelled emphatically at Dr. Miller as his head disappeared behind the OR door. He heard me. I didn't care. I grabbed one of my sterile gloves and slung it off my hand with a loud "thwack." My naked hand reached to the cuff of my other glove and with my thumb I pulled the stretchy latex edge of the glove away from me toward the trash can. The balled up gloves in my other hand were pulled back until they almost touched my face. I let the gloves go like a sling shot and they thumped against the far side of the can. Every nurse, even outside the OR, has shot their used gloves into the trash after using them. This time I pretended the gloves disintegrated against Dr. Miller's face. He was a total dick.

Seconds before, he had slammed open the OR door and demanded to know why I was delaying his case by putting in a foley for the patient he was about to operate on. Yes, the patient was asleep. "WHEN DID I SAY TO PUT A FOLEY IN?!? YOU ARE ALWAYS DELAYING ME FOR SOME SHIT!" This wasn't true, and it usually wasn't true for anyone else he flamed out on. My anger instantly reached near peak, but I slowly and tersely replied, "It's a fusion...it's booked for three hours...you always want a foley for fusions..." "THIS WILL ONLY TAKE 45 MINUTES!" he screamed. "Toss the foley and turn the patient." He muttered more expletives as he turned to walk out. As soon as the door closed, he popped his head back in and with an annoyed tone said, "well I'm trying something a little different for this one, maybe put one in after all..." I was still standing next to the stretcher with the foley kit before me, ready to insert and move on to the next task.

I was incensed that he couldn't just politely stop me like every other surgeon and simply say something like, "no thank you, that won't be necessary, this will be a much shorter procedure than a normal fusion so we won't need a foley." It was a newer procedure he had just started doing and whereas a traditional lumbar fusion might take 3-5 hours, this particular kind would only last one. No, he had to throw a hissy fit and literally stomp his feet like a child. He stood in the doorway and kept talking to himself whether or not he wanted a foley. "WHAT IS IT YOU WANT ME TO DO?!" My tone and volume matched his, surprising everyone in the room. After a second, Dr. Miller rebounded with a very definitive, "JUST FORGET IT!" as he turned to walk out. "FINE!"

I kicked the trash can out of my way and stepped over to the telephone on the wall. The scrub and CRNA looked at me from behind their masks with wide eyes. They both glanced beyond the OR door and back at me to try to see Dr. Miller out at the scrub sink. I punched in the phone number to call for positioning help. As the phone rang, I could feel my ears were hot. The surgeon took every chance he could to voice his displeasure at life. He was the kind of person to wish it was 70 degrees instead of 75 outside. He complained once that his Super Bowl seats weren't where he would have liked them. He spent the whole day voicing his regret he could only see half the game from the end zone. If Dr. Miller had gone down the hall to tell my manager a nurse had the nerve to yell at him, I really didn't care. For one thing, what I had done was reasonable considering the case was booked for three hours, and we always put in foleys for longer procedures like that. No one told me it would be shorter and I had no reason to think it would be. Plus, he swore at me and started the yelling in the first place. Besides, we were already short handed as it was since one nurse had just retired and another one had just switched to another specialty. I wasn't worried about "corrective action" from HR.

The OR techs and my coordinator came in the room a minute later to help turn the patient over onto the operating table. My usually talkative coordinator just looked at me without saying anything. She finally spoke. "Dr. Miller got a taste of his own medicine, huh?" She had been in the OR for twenty years, she knew what had happened. I angrily retold the encounter as we all took our places around the stretcher to roll the patient over onto the table. The scrub tech and CRNA chimed in defending me. My coordinator nodded as I went and let me finish. "Well, it's his birthday today so maybe that will bring him back to a better mood." I rolled my eyes.

A few minutes later, Dr. Miller came in the room uneventfully and began his own doctor's routine of looking at the x-rays on the wall computer and muttering to himself. He didn't acknowledge any of us or what had happened minutes earlier. A young pretty rep bounced in behind him seconds later. She had her iPad tucked under her arm and was hurriedly trying to tie her mask above her red bouffant hat. She awkwardly managed to finish and stepped next to Dr. Miller at the computer. They discussed the surgical plan and she readily and emphatically agreed with everything he said. I stood at my own computer charting with a fixed gaze. It had felt good to return fire at a surgeon. But now I wished to just do my work without any further interaction with him. I didn't want the awkward conversation of an apology(from him; I definitely wasn't sorry), or discussion about why I should have asked about the foley first. It would be okay, because neither of these things would happen.

The case started and actually went smoothly. Dr. Miller didn't complain about anything. He and the rep bantered throughout the case. The rep mentioned that it was Dr. Miller's birthday today and an awkward pause filled the room. Finally the scrub offered a "happy birthday." "I have a surprise for you in the break room when you're done Dr. Miller," the rep coyly said. About ten minutes from the end of the case, another nurse came in the room to give me lunch break. I told her the necessary things about the patient in the handoff report and walked out of the OR.

The first thing I saw when I walked into our small break room was a square Martin's cake box. This was the surprise for Dr. Miller. Everyone knew Martin's bakery. They were locally famous for their menu of twenty or so rotating cakes that they served throughout the year. They usually sold cakes by the slice from the counter, but of course also sold entire cakes. A regular whole cake was usually around $50. This one was a larger version and had to have been at least $75. I could see "Happy Birthday Dr. Miller!" written in big, cursive, frosted letters through the clear top window of the box. I could tell it was Martin's signature dark chocolate cake.

I was taking an early lunch, because that's the way it goes sometimes. No one else was in our small break room yet. I found a stack of foam takeout trays and took one. I sat it down on the table and opened the top of the cake box. Without a second thought I picked up the plastic serving knife that came with the cake and spun the cake around to where I planned to cut my wedge of cake out. I performed my own surgery right there in the break room with two wide lines, one above and below "Dr. Miller." The piece I cut was big enough for two people. I slid the knife under the heavy wedge and broke it away from the cake. I heard footsteps coming around the corner. I quickly plopped down the cake onto the plate. I was caught. The scrub tech came in and looked as though she had walked in on a murder. Chocolate cake crumbs and icing covered the knife in my hand. She said my name and exclaimed, "has Dr. Miller even seen his cake yet?" "Nope!" I replied. "Cut me a piece." I pointed to the stack of trays for her to grab one.

I closed my tray and hid it on top of the refrigerator for later. My accomplice hid her piece as well and left to go to the cafeteria. I closed the cake box and found my regular lunch. I walked over to the microwave and started warming up my meal. With my back turned, I heard someone else walk in. The rep opened the box and gasped, "Oh no! Who ate this already?!" She turned to look at me. "Did you cut this?" "No, just walked in." She was silently apoplectic. "I-I can't believe someone ate this already," she quietly spoke. I liked the rep, but I didn't feel bad. It would be just one more thing the doctor could complain about.

Chapter 4. Last Fight

Were my hands shaking? "Get a grip," I told myself. I moved onto my next question. "Do you have any metal implants in your body from past surgeries?", I asked the patient. "Yeah, broke my left arm when our truck rolled over in Baghdad. There a plate in there." I continued my interview. "Is this your wife?" "Yes, she's been mine for eight years." The young woman looked at me in a frozen stare, not blinking. She took a deep breath and her shoulders heaved. I could see her tears glistening as we briefly locked eyes. I couldn't look at her for more then a second. "Can we call her in the waiting room with updates during your case?" They both nodded yes. "Ok, well we will take good care of you sir, just another signature from Dr. Morgan and we will be on our way." I was relieved to be over with the conversation. The patient was my age, older than me by only a few weeks. He was young and in good shape. His wife clutched his hand and was visibly fighting back sobs. He laid on the stretcher calmly. I stepped to the other side of the holding room and waited for Dr. Morgan to visit the patient. The CRNA also joined me in a few minutes and grabbed a small tissue box that we gave out to patients or families when they needed one. "They are so strong" she said and I nodded in agreement. We shared a few comments between ourselves about the room set-up and other "shop talk." Anything we could talk about besides the young couple across the room. "I'll be right back," she said.

The surgeon had told me in the previous case that this patient was going to die in about six months, even after his brain tumor was removed. The brain surgery was only going to offer a little more time, the cancer was too aggressive to be completely stopped. The patient had been a soldier and came home to start a family and a business. He had two young children. When I was in nursing school, he had been in a far away desert getting shot at. This surgery would be his last battle.

Dr. Morgan emerged from the main OR hallway and saw me waiting at the corner where the holding room and hallway joined. He gave me a quick nod and walked over to the patient. There were six other patients lined up in a row, but he knew immediately which person to walk up to. The wife could not hold it in any more. She burst into a sob but soon collected herself as Dr. Morgan put his arm on her shoulder with one hand and grabbed the patient's arm with the other. They spoke for a few minutes and he then picked up the chart to sign his name. We looked at each other as he passed me. A quick nod and a deep exhale passed from Dr. Morgan as he quickly walked around the corner. We all could only maintain our composure for minutes at a time. The CRNA returned from where she had been and I motioned for her to wipe a streak of mascara from the side of her eye. "Did I get it?" I nodded yes. We had worked together for years, and she was glad I told her.

We both walked back over to the patient just in time for two little children to toddle into the holding room from the other hallway. The children and their grandmother walked straight over to the young man and his wife. The CRNA looked at me with huge eyes and gave my wrist a tight squeeze. I tapped her fist with two reassuring bumps and she let go. "Are these your kids? They're beautiful!", she gushed as the mother picked up the younger child. For a few seconds, the children's elation at seeing their parents distracted us from our own feelings about their Dad's prognosis. They kissed their Dad on the cheek. The mother held the younger child and stepped aside. The soldier's Mom planted a kiss on the top of her son's head and placed her hand on his chest. Her mouth stretched wide and tight across her face to also keep from crying. "Let's do it", he said.

As I kicked the lock pedal beneath the stretcher, it released with a loud click, jarring the emotional scene. "We'll take great care of him," I said like I always did when we departed the holding room. "We'll see you soon!", the CRNA said as she took her place behind the patient's head. I stood at the foot of the stretcher to guide it through the halls into the OR. The family began moving to the other side of the room as we began rolling away. The patient bit his upper lip hard and took a deep breath as soon as he was out of his family's sight. He had been strong for them and now I could tell he was also feeling the weight of the moment. As we turned into the hallway, the CRNA looked at me from the other side of the stretcher and waved her hand into her face as if to ward off more tears. The patient lied there between us and stared at the ceiling tiles passing above him. "Thank y'all for your help today."

We rolled into the room and it felt like any other case we had done before. The routine we knew so well took over and soon the heart wrenching scene we had witnessed earlier faded into the background of our minds. Moving the patient alongside the main table, locking the stretcher, helping him move over, securing the safety belt and arm boards. The CRNA also began her checklist of tasks to complete before the surgery began. Laying a warm blanket over the patient, rolling the stretcher back out into the hallway, walking over to the scrub to do our initial count. I could hear the CRNA tell the patient all the familiar things they tell everyone. "You'll be off to sleep soon, we will start another IV in this arm after you're asleep, pick out a good dream..."

What dream would he choose? Most people, if they said out loud what they picked, said they thought about their favorite beach or something else cliché. What does a man with less than a year to live think about before he goes to sleep? For a few minutes, all the ambient noises in the room coincidentally faded away except the steady beeping of the machine's pulse oximeter. The scrub stopped stacking the metal pans and arranging instruments. I stopped opening various supplies the surgeon would need later. We usually tried to get quiet anyway when the patient first went off the sleep, but this time the somber mood of the room created a stillness that I will always remember. The noisy OR would return in a few minutes.

Dr. Morgan came in the room without me calling him, like he always did. He had a knack for coming in right when it was his time. He didn't hover impatiently in the room before the patient came in, and he wasn't impossible to find after the patient had been positioned and ready for ten or more minutes. We positioned the patient and continued our routine. I popped the prep stick and waited as the cleaning solution flowed from its capsule inside the handle into the sponge applicator. I prepped the patient's head carefully; if a nurse wasn't mindful, the prep solution could run down into a patient's eye from the top of the head. When I was finished, I tapped the small egg timer velcroed to the wall to start the three minute countdown of the prep drying time. I returned to my computer and typed a few more things in the chart while Dr. Morgan scrubbed his hands and arms at the sink outside the room.

He came in, laughing at something someone said out in the hall. His arms were dripping water off his elbows as he walked over to the scrub. She handed him a sterile towel and opened his gown with a quick jerk as she shook it side to side. He was gowned and gloved and walked over to his patient. He and the scrub began unfolding and placing small blue towels and the large drape over our patient. Despite the unique circumstances this patient brought with him, after the drapes were on, the surgical field looked the same as any other under the bright lights. The scrub moved the tables and mayo stands around the room to the side of the patient as I waited for her to toss me the cords and suction tubing for me to connect. Dr. Morgan grabbed the sterile light handle covers and grabbed the lights above him, swiveling them to the right angle above the area he was about make an incision.

"Let's timeout." Patient name, date of birth, name of procedure, laterality, name of surgeon, duration, estimated blood loss, and anticipated specimens were all discussed. Dr. Morgan added, "let's give this soldier some more time with his family." For a brief time the somber mood returned but we carried on with our tasks. I flipped on the music system in our room to continue the surgical routine we knew so well. All of the familiar and expected things happened for the next two hours. The surgery itself was unremarkable. It was a good surgery, even if we all hated the ultimate outcome. At the end though, in addition to his typical "thanks everyone," before walking out of the room, Dr. Morgan stopped and told us how proud he was to work with us and thanked us for helping him. He said the family would be very appreciative of our work that day.

The CRNA and I took the man back out of the OR to the recovery room. He groggily acknowledged our voices as we spoke to him to re-orient him to the world. I wondered if as he became slowly aware he had momentarily forgotten his short time remaining on Earth. When bad things in my life happened like a car wreck or a family member passing away, for a minute or so after waking up the next day I didn't remember those things happening. Only after having my eyes open for a few seconds would those uncomfortable memories rush back in and make me want to go back to sleep. Perhaps everyday had been like that since the young man was told about his diagnosis. I hoped we had given him as much time remaining as we could.

I have no idea what my next case was. While the person receiving our care was just as valuable and unique as our soldier, they fell into the mass of people I've taken care of that all blend together after years and years of working in the OR. I do however remember the last three cases I had that day, which turned into a late night. I was on call, and as the normal cases in the OR finished around 7 pm, the phone at our desk rang. Dr. Morgan had an add-on. An emergency spine case. I groaned and began picking the case. An hour later, we were doing our timeout. Two hours later, we rolled the patient into recovery. By 10 pm, we were starting our next case, an emergency craniotomy for someone who had fallen and had a brain bleed. There was a new scrub and CRNA, but me and Dr. Morgan remained. "Long day, huh man!" he said to me with a smile as he came into the room from the scrub sink for the last time that day. With a groan, I replied, "you said it!" Another case, another patient ushered in and out of the OR. By now it was just after midnight.

I tossed my scrubs with authority into the linen basket in the locker room. I trudged out of the unit, down the main hall, onto the employee walkway to the parking deck. My car sat alone in the middle of the concrete, two white lines on either side. I remembered something our manager told us once in a staff meeting. In a thirty mile radius of our hospital, there were almost two million people. All those people would come to us in an emergency and at any time one of us in the OR would be called upon to use our skills. I felt the weight of that concept as I saw out of the hundred or so parking spots on my level, I was the only one remaining. The deck had been nearly full that morning as the work day started. I opened my car and turned on the heat. I was starving and tired, but awake. I stopped at a 24 hour diner on the way home and ordered a staple dinner of a burger and fries. By the end of the meal, I was very drowsy and tried to work myself into the mindset of staying awake fifteen more minutes for the drive home. I thought to myself how I needed to make more of an effort to give away my call.

Made in the USA
Columbia, SC
29 June 2023

19639403R00081